薬学生のための
英語会話

金子利雄・Eric M. Skier 編

English Conversation for Student Pharmacists

音声データダウンロードサービス付

東京化学同人

まえがき

　本書は，"薬学準備教育ガイドライン (3) 薬学の基礎としての英語 ③【聞く・話す】"
技能を養成するために開発された薬学英会話教材です．グローバル化が進む今日，薬剤師
が外国人患者・顧客に英語でコミュニケーションがとれることは，薬剤師という専門職に
とっての必須技能であり，"おもてなし"と"やさしさ"であると言えます．外国人患
者・顧客は薬剤師に救いの手を求めて医療機関にやってきます．そのような人たちを，英
語が苦手だから，話せないからという理由で，ぞんざいに扱うことは決してあってはなら
ないことです．薬剤師を志す皆さんは，このことをよく理解して，本書を活用して会話の
技能を修得していただくよう希望いたします．

　本書は，"薬学分野"を保険薬局，ドラッグストア，病院の三つの臨床現場に限定し，
それぞれの分野での代表的な Dialog を基本として取上げました．それを補助するものと
して，役に立つさまざまな表現をまとめた Useful Expressions，専門用語の正しい発音を
身につけるための Pronunciation Practice，Dialog の表現定着を再確認するための Speak
Like a Pharmacist in English，聴解力を確認するための Dictation，速読力を訓練するため
の Reading Comprehension，短い文章を聞き取り理解する Listening Comprehension，場
面に応じた対話を自ら作成する Make Your Own Dialog，各 Unit に関連する発展的な情報
を紹介する Column を取上げ，さらに薬剤師の活動の場を海外に求める高い志を抱く人た
ちのために米国・カナダの薬学教育事情，同一医薬品に用いられる英米の名称の違いなど
も加えました．

　本書は，2017-2019 学術研究助成基金助成金基盤研究（c），課題番号 17K02944 の成果
として，薬学生向けに編集した薬学英語会話教材です．本書を作成するにあたり，日本薬
学英語研究会（JAPE），ならびに所属大学，専門領域を問わず，多くの専門分野の先生方
の惜しみないご協力をいただきました．

　とりわけ，東京化学同人の住田六連氏と福富美保氏の薬学英語教育へのご理解とご支援
がなければ，本書は完成に至らなかったと思います．ここに深く感謝申し上げます．

　2021 年 1 月

"薬学生のための英語会話"編者・執筆者一同

執　筆　者

板 垣 　 正　　日本大学薬学部 専任講師, Ph.D. ［③(UNIT1〜15), ⑥(UNIT7)］*

井 原 久 美 子　昭和薬科大学薬学部 非常勤講師, 修士(薬学) ［⑥(UNIT12)］

岩 澤 真 紀 子　北里大学薬学部 講師, Pharm.D. ［①(UNIT11〜15), 海外の薬学教育・
薬剤師業務②］

金 子 利 雄　　日本大学薬学部 教授, 文学修士, M.A.(英語学) ［⑥(UNIT1, 4, 6, 15)］

河 野 享 子　　京都薬科大学薬学部 助教, 理学博士 ［⑥(UNIT5)］

齋 藤 弘 明　　日本大学薬学部 専任講師, 博士(薬学) ［⑥(UNIT8)］

Eric M. Skier　日本大学薬学部 准教授, M.A.(英語教授法) ［④(UNIT1〜15),
⑥(UNIT9, 11), ⑦(UNIT1〜15), 付表］

高 橋 和 子　　神奈川県立保健福祉大学保健福祉学部 講師, M.S.(医薬天然物化学),
修士(応用言語学), Ph.D.(免疫学) ［⑥(UNIT13)］

玉 巻 欣 子　　神戸薬科大学薬学部 教授, M.A.(応用言語学), 博士(医学) ［⑤(UNIT1〜15),
⑥(UNIT14)］

平 井 清 子　　北里大学一般教育部 教授, 修士(英語教育) ［⑥(UNIT3)］

堀 内 正 子　　昭和薬科大学薬学部 教授, 修士(英語教育) ［②(UNIT1〜15), ⑥(UNIT2)］

吉澤(渡邉)小百合　星薬科大学薬学部 准教授, 修士(教育学) ［⑥(UNIT10)］

渡 辺 朋 子　　前東邦大学薬学部 准教授, 博士(薬学) ［①(UNIT1〜10), 海外の薬学
教育・薬剤師業務①］

(五十音順)

* ［　］内は担当箇所： ① 冒頭の囲みと Dialog, ② Useful Expressions,
③ Pronunciation Practice, ④ Speak Like a Pharmacist in English, ⑤ Dictation,
⑥ Reading Comprehension と Listening Comprehension, ⑦ Make Your Own Dialog

コラム執筆者

安 部　　恵　　日本大学薬学部 准教授［UNIT9］

荒 川 基 記　　日本大学薬学部 専任講師，博士(薬学)［UNIT5］

泉 澤　　恵　　日本大学薬学部 専任講師，薬学修士，博士(医学)［UNIT4］

大 場 延 浩　　日本大学薬学部 教授，修士(医科学)，博士(薬学)［UNIT2］

小 野 真 一　　日本大学薬学部 教授，医学博士［UNIT15］

岸 川 幸生　　日本大学薬学部 教授，博士(医療薬学)［UNIT11］

辻　　泰 弘　　日本大学薬学部 教授，博士(薬学)［UNIT12］

中 島 理 恵　　日本大学薬学部 助教，修士(医科学)［UNIT6］

中 村 公薫　　日本大学薬学部 専任講師，修士(薬科学)［UNIT14］

中 山 敏 光　　日本大学医学部附属板橋病院臨床研究センター，博士(薬学)［UNIT13］

花 岡 峻 輔　　日本大学薬学部 助教［UNIT8］

林　　宏 行　　日本大学薬学部 教授，博士(薬学)［UNIT10］

日 髙 慎 二　　日本大学薬学部 教授，博士(薬学)［UNIT7］

福 岡 憲 泰　　日本大学薬学部 教授，博士(臨床薬学)，博士(医学)［UNIT1］

渡 邉 文 之　　日本大学薬学部 教授，博士(薬学)［UNIT3］

(五十音順，[ ] 内は担当箇所)

本書の使用にあたって

　本書は“薬学準備教育ガイドライン”で示された“(3) 薬学の基礎としての英語”の“薬学分野で必要とされる英語に関する基本的事項を修得する”という GIO に則り，“聞く・話す”能力に特化した英語会話教材である．薬学分野を，保険薬局，ドラッグストア，病院に限定し，そこで働く薬剤師に必要な英語会話スキルを養成することを目的とする．

　各 Unit は，冒頭の囲み，Dialog, Useful Expressions, Pronunciation Practice, Speak Like a Pharmacist in English, Dictation, Reading Comprehension, Listening Comprehension, Make Your Own Dialog, Column からなる．

　本書は，15 Unit からなるが，年 30 回の講義でも使用できるような十分な内容である．15 回の半期科目として使用する場合には，練習問題を適宜選択していただくことになる．担当教員は，ネイティブ，日本人のどちらでも本書を利用できるよう編集した．

　本書の使用方法は，次のとおりである．

【学生の方へ】

・囲み: 必ず読んで，Unit を始める前の予備知識を習得する．
・Dialog*: 音声を何度も聞いて，暗唱する．これが会話表現の基礎となる．
・Useful Expressions: 会話の基礎となるさまざまな医療表現，語彙を覚える．
・Pronunciation Practice*: 音声を聞いて正しい発音を身につける．
・Speak Like a Pharmacist in English: Dialog の表現定着を再確認する．
・Dictation[†]: 音声を聞いて書き取り，エラーの原因を考える．
・Reading Comprehension（本文*，質問[†]）: 音声を聞きながら読んで，内容を把握する．
・Listening Comprehension（本文*，質問*）: 音声のみを聞いて，質問に答える．
・Make Your Own Dialog: Dialog を思い出し，与えられた場面に合った対話文をつくる．
・Column: 各 Unit に関連した発展的情報を読み，知識を深める．
◆音声データは次ページの“ダウンロードの手順”に従ってダウンロードしてください．（＊印の音声が含まれます．†印の音声は授業の際に聞いてください．）

【担当の先生方へ】

　半期，通年のどちらでもご使用いただけるよう，Unit 数は 15 としながらも，問題量は豊富に用意しました．対象となる学生に応じた適切な進め方があるかと思います．臨床現場で必要となる会話表現の基本は，Dialog に集約されておりますので，この基本表現の定着を第一目標として，視覚と聴覚に訴えたレッスンが展開されることを願っております．また，Unit のほかに，学生の国際的視野を広げるために，海外での薬学事情を載せました．

◆教科書採用が確認された教員限定で，東京化学同人より教員用資料をお送りします．教員用資料には上記の＊印の音声に加えて，†印の音声が含まれます．†印の音声は学生には入手できませんので，授業の際に学生に聞かせてください．

🔊 音声データについて

音声データの内容

ファイル形式：MP3

録音内容：Dialog*，Pronunciation Practice*，Dictation†，Reading Comprehension（本文*，質問文†），Listening Comprehension（本文*，質問文*）

（＊印は学生用音声，教員用音声には＊印に加えて†印の音声が含まれます．）

録音時間：学生用音声 約 90 分，教員用音声 約 120 分

ナレーター：Eric M. Skier，Karen Haedrich

音声データダウンロードの手順・注意事項

MP3 形式の音声ファイルを ZIP 形式で提供いたします．下記の手順でダウンロードし，パソコンで再生してご利用ください．

[ダウンロードの手順]

1）パソコンで東京化学同人のホームページにアクセスし，書名検索などにより，"薬学生のための英語会話"の画面を表示させる．

2）画面最後尾の 音声ダウンロード をクリックし，下記のユーザー名およびパスワードを入力する．（本書購入者本人以外は使用できません．図書館での利用は館内での使用に限ります．）

ユーザー名：**MjB58rf9**

パスワード：**26PuWT5m**

[サインイン] を選択すると，ダウンロードが始まる．

※ ファイルは ZIP 形式で圧縮されていますので，解凍ソフトで解凍のうえ，ご利用ください．

[必要な動作環境]

音声データのダウンロードおよび再生には，下記の動作環境を推奨します．この動作環境を満たしていないパソコンでは正常にダウンロードおよび再生ができない場合がありますので，ご了承ください．

OS：Microsoft Windows 10，Mac OS X, 11（日本語版サービスパックなどは最新版）

推奨ブラウザ：Microsoft Edge，Microsoft Internet Explorer，Safari など

コンテンツ再生：Microsoft Windows Media Player 12，Quick Time Player など

［**音楽 CD プレイヤーで再生するには**］

　音楽 CD プレイヤーなどで再生する場合には，パソコン上で適切なアプリケーション（Windows Media Player12 など）を用いて，オーディオ CD（データ CD ではない）を作成していただく必要があります．CD は 1 枚では入りきらないので 2 枚ご準備ください．オーディオ CD の作成の仕方は，各アプリケーションの説明書でご確認ください．弊社でのお客様ごとの個別対応はいたしかねますのでご了承ください．

［**データ利用上の注意**］

・本音声データのダウンロードおよび再生に起因して使用者に直接または間接的障害が生じても株式会社東京化学同人はいかなる責任も負わず，一切の賠償などは行わないものとします．

・本音声データの全権利は権利者が保有しています．本音声データのいかなる部分についても，データバンクへの取込みを含む一切の電子的，機械的複製および配布，送信を，書面による許可なしに行うことはできません．許可を求める場合は，東京化学同人（東京都文京区千石 3-36-7，info@tkd-pbl.com）にご連絡ください．

目　　次

イラスト：ふくとみあやこ

PART I

Community Pharmacy

UNIT 1

Drop Off:
Filling a Prescription

薬局は，医療保険制度のなかの一施設であり，薬剤師が医師の処方箋に基づき調剤を行い，医薬品の販売または授与をする医療提供施設である．日本の医療保険制度は，すべての国民が何らかの公的医療保険に加入する国民皆保険制度を採用しており，医療サービスは健康保険で行われる．一部を除き，医療費の 70％ が公的医療保険から支払われる．健康保険による診療で交付された処方箋薬の費用も公的医療保険により支払われる．日本では，外国人居住者も日本の健康保険に加入することになるため，健康保険を取得している外国人居住者の医療費もその 70％ は公的医療保険で支払われる．一方で，日本の健康保険をもたない訪日外国人が日本で医療サービスを受けた場合には，医療費の全額を支払わなければならない．したがって，処方箋による調剤を希望する患者には，国籍に関わらず，健康保険証の確認をする必要がある．

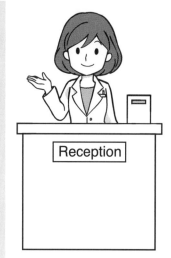

Reception

1・1　Dialog

■ Listen to the dialog and memorize it.

Track 1

[患] Excuse me, can I get this prescription filled here?

[薬] May I see it, please?

[患] Here you are.

[薬] Thank you. Is this your first time here?

[患] Yes, it is.

[薬] Do you have a Japanese health insurance card?

[患] Yes, I do.

[薬] Could you show me your card?

[患] Here you go.

[薬] Thank you very much. Please have a seat until your prescription is ready.

患: 患者
薬: 薬剤師

prescription 処方箋（処方箋薬）

Japanese health insurance card 健康保険証

患 How long will it take?

薬 It should take about 15 minutes. We will call your name when it is ready.

患 Okay.

1・2　Useful Expressions

■ Let's learn how to describe *types of physical conditions and lifestyles*：

(1) I have _____Ⓐ_____.

　　Ⓐ：atopy（アトピー）

　　　　a sensitive stomach（胃が弱い）

　　　　snacks between meals（間食）

　　　　stiffness in my shoulders or neck（肩や首がこる）

(2) I suffer from _____Ⓑ_____.

　　Ⓑ：nasal inflammation（鼻炎）

　　　　sensitivity to cold（冷え性）

　　　　hay fever/a pollen allergy（花粉症）

(3) I often get _____Ⓒ_____.（〜しやすい）

　　Ⓒ：diarrhea（下痢）　　constipated（便秘になった）　　convulsions（痙攣）

　　　　rashes from skin patches（貼り薬でかぶれやすい）

(4) I take _____Ⓓ_____.

　　Ⓓ：dietary supplements（健康食品）　　vitamins

　　　　snacks between meals（間食）

(5) I drink _____Ⓔ_____.

　　Ⓔ：beer　　　　sake　　　　shochu　　　　whisky　　　　wine

(6) I smoke _____Ⓕ_____.

　　Ⓕ：half a pack a day（1日に半箱たばこを吸う）　　a pipe（パイプを吸う）

(7) I drive a car/a motorcycle _____Ⓖ_____.

　　Ⓖ：every day　　once a week　　twice a week　　three times a week

(8) I feel very tired these days.（最近疲れがひどい）

Work in Pairs

One partner asks about physical conditions or lifestyle. His/her partner tries to explain the problems from (1)−(8) on page 4. Change roles.

Example
Ⓐ May I ask you about your physical condition?
Ⓑ Yes, I often get diarrhea.

Answers:

Ⓐ _____

Ⓑ _____

1·3 Pronunciation Practice

■ Pronounce the following words with special emphasis on accent, rhythm, and stress, etc... ◀))) Track 2

1. prescription
   [priskrípʃən]
2. insurance
   [inʃú(ə)rəns]
3. aspirin
   [ǽspərin]
4. herb
   [ə́ːrb]
5. stomach
   [stʌ́mək]
6. pharmacy
   [fɑ́rməsi]
7. ache
   [éik]
8. allergy
   [ǽlərdʒi]
9. vitamin
   [váitəmin]

1·4 Speak Like a Pharmacist in English

■ Answer the following questions orally in English.

Questions:

1. Ask a patient to show you her prescription.

_____

2. Ask a patient if she has Japanese health insurance.

_____

3. Ask the patient to show you her health insurance card.

_____

4. What is a polite way to tell a patient to wait?

_____

5. What will you say to tell a patient when her prescription is ready?

_____

1・5   Dictation

■ Listen carefully and write down what is said.

教のマークの音声は
学生用音声データに
含まれていません.
教室で聞いて下さい.

Answers:

1. _____

2. _____

3. _____

4. _____

5. _____

6. _____

7. _____

8. _____

1・6   Reading Comprehension

 Track 4

■ Read the following passage within 5 minutes and answer all the questions orally in English.

The prescription process starts in the doctor's office or at the health clinic. Tell the doc if you're taking any medicines — even over-the-counter（OTC）medicines like vitamins or herbal medicines. With some medicines, there's a risk that one might cause problems with the other（known in the medical profession as an interaction）.

For example, certain prescription medicines can make birth control pills less effective. Speaking of birth control, your doc will probably ask about birth control or whether you use alcohol or illegal drugs. It may seem awkward to talk about these topics, but your doc needs to know if you've taken anything that might interact with the prescription medicine. Don't worry, though — your doctor isn't there to judge you or report back to your parents.

Many doctors find ·a way to speak privately with teen patients so they can share confidential information. So don't hesitate to talk openly.

出 典: *How to Fill a Prescription*, KidsHealth のウエブサイト〔https://kidshealth.org/ en/teens/rx-filled.html?WT.ac=ctg（2019 年 11 月現在）〕より転載. © 1995-2019. The Nemours Foundation/KidsHealth®. All Rights Reserved.

Questions（Listen to the recording.）

Answers：

1. _____

2. _____

3. _____

4. _____

5. _____

6. _____

1 · 7   Listening Comprehension

 Track 6   ■ Listen carefully and answer all the questions orally in English.

Questions:

1. If you don't want to ask something personal in front of others, what can you choose to do?
2. When you have questions but don't want to ask them in the pharmacy, what can you say?
3. Where does useful information on dosages come from?
4. What does the useful information tell you?
5. If you don't feel well after taking a medicine, what should you do?
6. What can your pharmacist do for you?

Answers:

1. _____

2. _____

3. _____

4. _____

5. _____

6. _____

1 · 8   Make Your Own Dialog

■ Based on what you studied in this unit, work with a partner to make a dialog in English between a pharmacist and a patient.

Situation

　　　A foreign patient is visiting a pharmacy where you are on clinical rotation. The patient has brought a prescription from the U.S. This patient does not have Japanese health insurance. Provide information to the patient on how to get the medicine.

Answers：

A _____

B _____

A _____

B _____

A _____

B _____

A _____

B _____

COLUMN　　　処方箋受付（健康保険証の確認，海外の処方箋）

　保険薬局において保険調剤を受付ける場合，以下のようなことを行わなければなりません．まず，患者から健康保険証を提示してもらい，基礎情報（氏名，生年月日，性別，被保険者証の記号番号，住所，必要に応じて緊急連絡先）によって患者が療養の給付を受ける資格を有することを確認します．処方箋は使用期間が交付日を含めて4日以内とされている（長期の旅行など特殊な場合を除く）ので，処方日とともに保険医療機関名，処方医師氏名，処方内容および調剤内容について確認します．処方箋に記載されている番号が間違っていたり，保険資格を喪失していたりする

と，あとから患者が薬代を支払わなければならないといった手間がかかることにもなります．処方箋は国内で発行されたものに限るので，海外の処方箋については受付けることはできません．以上のことに併せて，お薬手帳についても持っているかどうかを尋ねます．この手帳には，患者の過去から現在まで処方された薬について書いてあります．相互作用の発現や同じ薬が別の診療科から処方される重複処方を防ぐことに役立つので，手帳の活用は薬による安全な治療を行うことにつながります．　　　　　　　　　　　　　　　（福岡憲泰）

UNIT 2

Drop Off: Patient Questionnaire

　薬剤師は，処方箋に基づく調剤を行うだけでなく，患者に適切な薬物療法を提供する役割を担っている．すなわち，薬の重複投与，相互作用（薬物−薬物，薬物−食物，薬物−疾患など），薬物アレルギーおよび有害作用を防ぎ，患者に安全で効果的な薬物療法を提供する責務がある．その役割を果たすため，事前に患者のアレルギーおよび副作用の有無，服薬状況，既往歴，現在の病状，一般用医薬品（OTC 医薬品）および健康食品の使用状況，生活習慣などの情報をアンケート調査により入手し，不適切な薬物療法を防ぐことが必要である．

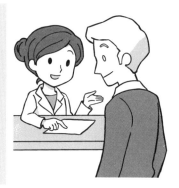

2・1　Dialog

 Track 7　■ Listen to the dialog and memorize it.

患 Hello. I would like to get this prescription filled?

薬 Have you been here before?

患 No, this is my first time here.

薬 Do you have time?

患 Yes, I do.

questionnaire アンケート，質問表

薬 We would like you to fill out this questionnaire.

患 Why do I need to fill out this survey in a pharmacy? I've already done a questionnaire at the hospital.

duplicate medications 重複薬

薬 We use it to check duplicate medications, drug interactions, side effects, etc. The information you share will help us to provide you with a safe and effective drug therapy.

患 OK, I understand.

薬 We appreciate your understanding.

患 (After completing the questionnaire) Here you go.

薬 Thank you very much. Please wait a few minutes until your prescription is ready.

患　Can I come back later?

薬　Yes, you can.　When you return, please give your name and show your number ticket at the pick-up counter.

患　Okay.　I'll be back in a little while.

2・2　Useful Expressions

■ Let's learn how to describe *symptoms*：pain

(1) I have ＿＿＿Ⓐ＿＿＿.

Ⓐ：a pain here （ここが痛い）

a headache （頭痛）　　　　　　　a slight headache （軽い頭痛）

a throbbing headache （ズキンズキンとする頭痛）

a frontal headache （額のあたりが重く痛い）

a severe/bad/terrible headache （ものすごい・がまんできない頭痛）

a stomachache （胃が痛い）　　　　abdominal pain （お腹が痛い）

epigastric pain （みぞおち付近が痛む）　side pain （脇腹が痛い）

hunger pains （空腹時にお腹が痛む）　chest pain （胸が痛い）

lower back pain/a backache （腰痛）　a sore throat （喉が痛い）

pain in the ear/an earache （耳が痛い）　a toothache （歯が痛い）

heartburn （キリキリするような疝痛がある）

pain in my big toe （足の親指の付け根が痛い）

pain in the finger joint/arthralgia （指の関節が痛い）

muscle pain/myalgia （筋肉痛がある）

pain when I urinate/pain when I pee （排尿痛がある）

my period/menstrual pain （生理痛がある）

(2) I feel ＿＿＿Ⓑ＿＿＿.

Ⓑ：chest pain　　　　　　　　sore all over from working out

pain in my shoulder

(3) My finger is arthritic. （指の関節が痛い）

My eyes hurt.

My heart is broken.

My headache is killing me.

Work in Pairs

One partner asks about physical conditions. His/her partner tries to name a few symptoms from (1) – (3) on page 11. Change roles.

Example

A What's wrong?

B I have a headache.

Answers:

A _____

B _____

2・3   Pronunciation Practice

))) Track 8

■ Pronounce the following words with special emphasis on accent, rhythm, and stress, etc...

1. questionnaire
   [kwèstʃənèər]

2. abdominal
   [æbdɑ́mənl]

3. muscular
   [mʌ́skjulər]

4. symptom
   [símptəm]

5. hygiene
   [háidʒiːn]

6. therapy
   [θérəpi]

7. appreciate
   [əpríːʃièit]

8. severe
   [səvíər]

9. duplicate
   [djúːplikət] （形容詞）

2・4   Speak Like a Pharmacist in English

■ Answer the following questions orally in English.

Questions:

1. How do you ask a patient if this is his first time to your drugstore?

2. How do you ask a patient to fill out a patient survey?

_____

3. How do you ask if they have time to fill out a survey?

_____

4. Explain why you are asking the patient to fill out a patient survey.

_____

5. Tell a patient the procedure for returning later to pick up a prescription.

_____

_____

2・5 Dictation

■ Listen carefully and write down what is said.   教))Track 9

Answers:

1. _____

2. _____

3. _____

4. _____

5. _____

6. _____

7. _____

8. _____

2・6   Reading Comprehension

 Track 10   ■ Read the following passage within 5 minutes and answer all the questions orally in English.

Depression is more than simply feeling unhappy or fed up for a few days. Most people go through periods of feeling down, but when you're depressed you feel persistently sad for weeks or months, rather than just a few days.

Some people think depression is trivial and not a genuine health condition. They're wrong — it is a real illness with real symptoms. Depression is not a sign of weakness or something you can "snap out of" by "pulling yourself together".

The good news is that with the right treatment and support, most people with depression can make a full recovery.

出 典: *Clinical Depression*, NHS のウエブサイト〔https://www.nhs.uk/conditions/clinical-depression/(2019 年 11 月現在)〕より転載. © Crown copyright

 Track 11   **Questions**（Listen to the recording.）

Answers：

1.

2.

3.

4.

5.

6.

2・7　Listening Comprehension

■ Listen carefully and answer all the questions orally in English.)) Track 12

Questions:

1. In which kind of foods are sugars found naturally?

2. To which kinds of foods are sugars added?

3. Which types of sugary foods do we need to cut down on?

4. Why should we decrease regular consumption of foods and drinks high in sugar?

5. What do nutrition labels tell us about sugar?

6. How can we make use of nutrition labels?

Answers:

1. _____

2. _____

3. _____

4. _____

5. _____

6. _____

2・8　Make Your Own Dialog

■ Based on what you studied in this unit, work with a partner to make a dialog in English between a pharmacist and a patient.

Situation

　　A patient who has a problem with his vision visits a pharmacy where you are on a clinical rotation. This is his first visit to your pharmacy. Ask him about his medications and lifestyle.

Answers:

A _____

B _____

A _____

B _____

A _____

B _____

A _____

B _____

COLUMN

初回来局時のアンケート

　初回来局時のアンケートは，薬剤師が患者の健康の維持や増進をサポートするために必要な情報を収集することが目的です．現在治療中の疾病や既往，処方された薬以外の薬，食べ物や薬によるアレルギーや副作用歴，お酒やたばこなどの嗜好品の摂取状況，サプリメントの使用，仕事や生活状況，後発医薬品の希望に関する情報を取得します．薬を管理する家族がいるか確認することもあります．

　たとえば，脳梗塞の予防に抗凝固薬（ワルファリン）が処方された場合，薬の効果を確認しながら投与されるので投与量が変更になる可能性があります．また，ときには納豆を食べることによる薬の効果減弱を避けながら，薬による疾病の管理に関与していきます．車の運転を職業としている場合，眠気が生じる薬は避けなければなりません．潰瘍治療薬の処方が出された患者がヘビースモーカーの場合，喫煙が潰瘍のリスクを増加することを理解してもらう必要があります．高齢の男性が鼻水を抑えるために抗ヒスタミン作用のある薬を服用すると，それが抗コリン作用を併せもつ場合，尿が出にくくなります．このように，初回来局時に薬や病気に関する情報を把握することが，患者の適切な薬物療法の実践につながります．　　　　　　　　　（大場延浩）

UNIT 3

Explaining: Contents and Directions

患者に安全で効果的な薬物療法を提供するためには，患者が薬物療法を理解し，調剤した薬を適切に服用する必要がある．そのために薬剤師は，患者に適正な情報を提供する必要がある．薬剤師法第25条には，"薬剤師は，調剤した薬剤の適正な使用のため，販売又は授与の目的で調剤したときは，患者又は現にその看護に当たつている者に対し，必要な情報を提供し，及び必要な薬学的知見に基づく指導を行わなければならない"と規定されており，適正な情報提供は薬剤師の責務である．

さらに，患者が提供した情報を理解し，アドヒアランスを向上させるために，専門用語ではなく一般的な言葉を使用して患者が情報を容易に理解できるようにしなければならない．

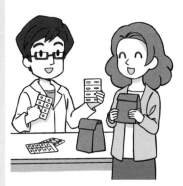

3・1 Dialog

■ Listen to the dialog and memorize it. ◀)) Track 13

薬 Mrs. Smith, sorry to have kept you waiting.

患 That's all right.

薬 You have three kinds of medicines today. This is the same medicine as last time. It helps lower your blood pressure. Please take one tablet at a time, once a day, after breakfast. This is for four weeks.

blood pressure
血圧

患 Okay. What are these two medicines for?

薬 What did your doctor tell you about your medicines?

患 She told me that she would prescribe some medicines for my cold.

prescribe 処方する

薬 All right. This packet is for the common cold. This medicine relieves several cold symptoms. And this medicine reduces throat swelling and pain from inflammation. Take one of each, three times daily, after each

relieve 緩和する

throat swelling
喉の腫れ

meal. These are for five days.

患 I see.

薬 This medicine may make you drowsy. Do not drive a car or operate machinery after you take it.

患 I understand. Thank you.

薬 I hope you feel better soon.

3・2   Useful Expressions

■ Let's learn how to describe *symptoms*： cold

(1) I have ＿＿＿＿Ⓐ＿＿＿＿.

　　　Ⓐ： a fever（熱）　　　　　　　a high fever/temperature（高熱）

　　　　　 a slight fever（微熱）　　　chills with a headache（頭痛を伴う寒気）

　　　　　 dizziness（めまい, ふらつき） a runny/running nose（鼻水）

　　　　　 diarrhea（下痢）　　　　　a dry cough at night（夜中に空咳）

　　　　　 a cough and yellowish sputum（咳と黄色っぽい痰）

　　　　　 diarrhea four times a day（1 日 4 回も水溶性下痢）

　　　　　 severe vomiting and diarrhea（吐きくだしがひどい）

(2) I am ＿＿＿＿Ⓑ＿＿＿＿.

　　　Ⓑ： sneezing a lot（しばしばくしゃみをする）

　　　　　 nauseous（吐き気を催す, むかむかする）

(3) I feel ＿＿＿＿Ⓒ＿＿＿＿.

　　　Ⓒ： febrile（熱っぽい）   sick（気分が悪い）   nauseous

　　　　　 cold（寒気がする）   chilly（肌寒い）   dull/sluggish（活気のない）

　　　　　 dizzy（目がまわる）   like vomiting/throwing up（吐き気がする）

(4) My temperature is above 38℃.（体温が 38℃ 以上ある）

(5) I have got/caught a cold.（かぜをひき現在もひいている）

(6) I may have the flu.（インフルエンザにかかったらしい）

Work in Pairs

One partner asks about physical conditions. His/her partner tries to name a few symptoms from (1) – (6) on page 18. Change roles.

Example

A What's wrong?

B My temperature is above 38℃. I may have the flu.

Answers：

A _____

B _____

3・3 Pronunciation Practice

■ Pronounce the following words with special emphasis on accent, rhythm, and stress, etc...   ))) Track 14

1. diarrhea
   [dàiəríːə]

2. medication
   [mèdəkéiʃən]

3. throat
   [θróut]

4. relieve
   [rilíːv]

5. inflammation
   [ìnfləméiʃən]

6. tablet
   [tǽblit]

7. drowsy
   [dráuzi]

8. swallow
   [swάlou]

9. blood
   [blʌ́d]

3・4 Speak Like a Pharmacist in English

■ Answer the following questions orally in English.

Questions：

1. Apologize to a patient for having made her wait.

2. Tell a patient how many medicines are in her prescription.

_____

3. Tell her how to take a medicine that lowers blood pressure.

_____

4. Reconfirm with a patient about her meds and what the doctor told her.

_____

5. Tell a patient a precaution about her medication.

_____

3・5   Dictation

教)) Track 15   ■ Listen carefully and write down what is said.

Answers:

1. _____

2. _____

3. _____

4. _____

5. _____

6. _____

7. _____

8. _____

3・6   Reading Comprehension

■ Read the following passage within 5 minutes and answer all the questions Track 16
orally in English.

> The strength of a medicine is the amount of active ingredient i.e. the drug that it contains. The strength of a medicine does not have anything to do with the size of a tablet/capsule or the amount of a liquid! Some medicines are prescribed as 'PRN,' which means 'as required.' An example is painkillers, which may be prescribed for use only when a client actually feels pain and not regularly taken. It is important to stick to the minimum time interval and the maximum daily doses when giving PRN medication. Some medicines need to be taken at specific times to work their best. For example, some antibiotics must be taken on an empty stomach as food reduces the drug availability. Some anti-inflammatory medicines need to be taken with or after food to reduce the chances of causing stomach problems.

出 典： 4. Strength, Dosage, Timing and Frequency of Medicines, Pharmacy Xpress のウ エブサイト〔http://www.pharmacy-xpress.co.uk/manuals/training-handbook/4-strength-dosage-timing-and-frequency-medicines（2019 年 11 月 現 在)〕 より転載. © Pharmacy Xpress 2013.

Questions（Listen to the recording.）

Answers：

1. _____

2. _____

3. _____

4. _____

5. _____

6. _____

3 · 7   Listening Comprehension

🔊)) Track 18   ■ Listen carefully and answer all the questions orally in English.

Questions:

1. What are the important aspects of medication adherence?
2. Why do we need to take our medication as prescribed?
3. What percentage of chronic disease treatment failures, per year, are caused by medication non-adherence?
4. How many chronic disease patients in America die because of non-adherence per year?
5. Which institution provided the above information?
6. What are statins most commonly used for?

Answers:

1. _____

2. _____

3. _____

4. _____

5. _____

6. _____

3 · 8   Make Your Own Dialog

■ Based on what you studied in this unit, work with a partner to make a dialog in English between a pharmacist and a patient.

Situation

Mr. Brown brought a prescription to the pharmacy where you are on a clinical rotation. The contents of the prescription are as follows:

Rp1. Adalat CR 20 mg one tablet at a time, once a day, after
breakfast, for 28 days
Rp2. PL granule Loxonin 60 mg one at a time, three times a day,
after each meal, for five days

Instruct him on how to take the medicines and provide him with drug
information.

Answers:

A _____

B _____

A _____

B _____

A _____

B _____

A _____

B _____

| COLUMN | 認知再構成法とは？ |

　薬局に来局する患者のなかには薬剤師の伝える知識や情報（服薬指導）を受け取る準備ができていない人がいます．そのような人にはまず，心に寄り添いながら患者が抱えている問題を解決する，または気持ちを楽にしてあげる必要があります．そんなとき**認知再構成法**が役に立ちます．認知再構成法は認知行動療法のスキルの一つです．認知行動療法とは，“人間の気分や行動が認知のあり方（ものの考え方・受け取り方）に影響を受ける”という理解に基づき構造化された精神療法です．そして認知再構成法は，考え方のクセにしばられて問題解決が進んでいないときに活用でき

るスキルです．認知再構成法を用いた患者支援では，不安な出来事などが起こったとき，患者の頭に浮かんだ考えをとらえ，気分などを確認したうえで，その考えを裏づける事実（根拠）とその考えと矛盾する事実（患者が気づいていない事実：反証）を薬剤師の問いかけにより，患者自身が自ら気づくよう導くことで，患者に視野を広げた考えをもってもらい，その結果として，考え方が適応的（適応的思考）になり気分が楽になる，というものです．このスキルを身につけるとワンランク上の患者支援が行えるようになるはずです．

（渡邉文之）

UNIT 4

Generic Medicine

　後発医薬品（ジェネリック医薬品）とは，先に開発された先発医薬品（新薬）の有効成分の特許が切れた後に製造された医薬品である．先発医薬品と同一の有効成分を同一量含み，同一の経路から投与する製剤で，効果・効能，用法・用量が原則的に同一で，先発医薬品と同等の臨床効果・作用が得られるとして，厚生労働省から認可されている．研究開発に要する費用が低く抑えられることから，先発医薬品よりも薬価が安くなる．日本の国民医療費は年々増加し続けており，後発医薬品の使用は，医療費を抑えるための解決策の一つである．さらに，患者の経済的な負担の軽減にもなることから，国は後発医薬品の使用を促進している．

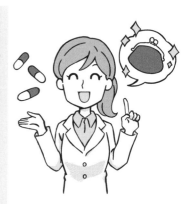

4・1　Dialog

 Track 19　■ Listen to the dialog and memorize it.

薬 Mr. David Hudson?

患 Here I am.

薬 Your prescription has been changed today and this prescription is available as a generic medicine. Would you mind trying a generic medicine?

generic medicine
後発医薬品

患 What is a generic medicine?

active ingredient
有効成分

薬 Generic medicines have the same active ingredients as branded medicines, but they are less expensive.

branded medicine
先発医薬品

患 Are the effects the same as those of the branded medicines?

薬 Yes, generic medicines are made to have the same effects as branded medicines.

患 Are they safe?

薬 Yes, they are. All generic medicines sold in Japan must be approved by the Japanese Ministry of Health, Labour and Welfare.

患 I understand. I'll take it.

薬 OK. Now please have a seat until your prescription is ready.

4・2　Useful Expressions

■ Let's learn how to describe *symptoms*: eye, ear, nose, throat*1

*1 耳鼻咽喉科医をENT doctorとよぶ.

(1) I have _____Ⓐ_____.

　　Ⓐ: blurred vision（かすみ目）　　　double vision（物が二重に見える）

　　　　watery eyes（涙目）　　　　　irritated eyes（目がごろごろする）

　　　　red eyes（目の充血）　　　　　itchy eyes（目のかゆみ）

　　　　earwax（耳垢）　　　　　　　tinnitus（耳鳴り）

　　　　a very painful eye and continuous tears（目が痛くて涙がいっぱい出る）

　　　　a throbbing pain in my left ear（左の耳がズキズキ痛む）

　　　　a pain in my ear after swimming（泳いだ後耳が痛い）

　　　　a blocked and runny nose（鼻が詰まって鼻水が多い）

　　　　a frontal headache with nasal congestion（鼻が詰まって額が重苦しくて痛い）

　　　　violent sneezing fits（くしゃみがひどい）

　　　　a sore throat with difficulty swallowing（喉が痛くて物が飲み込みにくい）

(2) I feel something strange _____Ⓑ_____.（異物感がある）

　　Ⓑ: in my eye　　in my ear　　in my nose

(3) My eyes are _____Ⓒ_____.

　　Ⓒ: sore（痛い）　　burning（焼けるように痛い）　　very itchy（とても痒い）

(4) My throat is _____Ⓓ_____.

　　Ⓓ: very irritated（とてもいがらっぽい）　　scratchy（少しヒリヒリする）
　　　　full of phlegm（痰が詰まる）

(5) I am sneezing a lot.（よくくしゃみをする）

(6) I've got*2 hearing loss after tuberculosis therapy.（結核治療で難聴になった.）

*2 have, have got はしばしば同義で使われる.

Work in Pairs

One partner asks about physical conditions. His/her partner tries to name a few symptoms from (1)–(6) on page 25. Change roles.

Example
A What's wrong?
B I have a sore throat with difficulty swallowing.

Answers:

A _____

B _____

4・3   Pronunciation Practice

)) Track 20   ■ Pronounce the following words with special emphasis on accent, rhythm, and stress, etc...

1. tuberculosis
   [tjubə̀ːrkjulóusis]

2. ingredient
   [ingríːdiənt]

3. generic
   [dʒənérik]

4. glucose
   [glúːkous]

5. pneumonia
   [njumóunjə]

6. asthma
   [ǽzmə]

7. pollen
   [pálən]

8. protein
   [próutiːn]

9. insulin
   [ínsəlin]

4・4   Speak Like a Pharmacist in English

■ Answer the following questions orally in English.

Questions:

1. Tell a patient that a generic form of a medicine exists.

_____

2. Ask the patient if he prefers a branded medicine or a generic form.

_____

In the United States, 9 out of 10 prescriptions filled are for generic drugs. Increasing the availability of generic drugs helps to create competition in the marketplace, which then helps to make treatment more affordable and increases access to healthcare for more patients.

The FDA's Office of Generic Drugs (OGD) within the Center for Drug Evaluation in Research ensures that people have access to safe, affordable generic drugs by following a rigorous review process that includes:

- Managing the regulatory process to facilitate drug approvals,
- Establishing science initiatives to research generic drugs,
- Publishing data and reports on generic drug development and review, and
- Offering educational materials and information.

出 典: *Generic Drugs*, U.S. FDA のウエブサイト〔https://www.fda.gov/drugs/buying-using-medicine-safely/generic-drugs（2019 年 11 月現在)〕より転載.

Questions（Listen to the recording.）

Answers:

1. _____

2. _____

3. _____

4. _____

5. _____

6. _____

4・7 Listening Comprehension

■ Listen carefully and answer all the questions orally in English. Track 24

Questions:

1. When can you introduce generic drugs?
2. How long does a drug patent last in principle?
3. Why are generic drugs available at a lower cost?
4. What do you do when you want to lower what you pay at the pharmacy?
5. Which patient would not financially benefit from a generic medicine?
6. Who can benefit significantly from a change to a generic medicine?

Answers:

1. _____

2. _____

3. _____

4. _____

5. _____

6. _____

4・8 Make Your Own Dialog

■ Based on what you studied in this unit, work with a partner to make a dialog in English between a pharmacist and a patient.

Situation

A patient brought a prescription to the pharmacy where you are on a clinical rotation. The prescription is available to be changed to a generic medicine. Ask him if he would mind changing to a generic medicine. And explain to him about generic medicines.

Answers:

A _____

B _____

A _____

B _____

A _____

B _____

A _____

B _____

COLUMN

後 発 医 薬 品

　後発医薬品とは，先に開発・販売されてきた "先発医薬品（新薬）" に対し，先発医薬品の特許が切れた後で製造された医薬品です．新薬の再審査期間と特許権存続期間の両方が満了すると，新薬と同じ有効成分の医薬品を "後発医薬品（ジェネリック医薬品）" として他の製薬企業が製造・販売することが可能になるからです．後発医薬品を製造・販売する際には，厚生労働省から製造販売承認を取得することが必要となります．大事な要件は，"先発医薬品と同等の品質"，"生物学的同等性が確保されていること" であり，これを科学的に証明した資料などが必要になります．生物学的同等性試験を行う目的は，先発医薬品に対する後発医薬品の科学的な同等性を保証することにあり，相対的なバイオアベイラビリティを比較することになります．

　後発医薬品販売の 2020 年の政府目標は，数量 80％であり，目標到達は間近になってきましたが，現状ではその利益の確保が難しく一つの節目を迎えます．2020 年度には，薬価基準の価格改定が一本化され，毎年の薬価改定がスタートします．今後，後発医薬品メーカーの課題は，競争を生き抜く独自の存在価値が求められていくことです．　　　　　　　　　　　　　　　　（泉澤　恵）

UNIT 5

At the Cashier

UNIT 1 で述べたとおり，日本の医療保険制度では，原則として医療サービスでかかった費用の70％は公的医療保険から支払われるが，残りの30％は一部負担金として患者自身が支払わなければならない．薬局も医療制度のなかの一施設であることから，薬局の調剤でかかった費用の30％は患者自身が支払うことになる．現在，世界はキャッシュレスの傾向にあり，海外では電子マネーによる支払いが進んでいるが，日本ではいまだに現金での支払いが主流となっている．特に医療機関では，クレジットカードでの支払いを受け付けない機関が多く，現金での支払いを余儀なくされる．薬局でも現金での支払いを求めるところが多い．

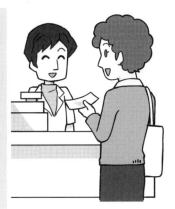

5・1 Dialog

■ Listen to the dialog and memorize it.

 Track 25

薬 Ms. Susan Smith?

患 Yes, that's me.

薬 Your medicines will come to 4,560 yen.

患 I have a Japanese health insurance card and I can't understand why I need to pay so much for my medicine. I don't need to pay any medical costs at a pharmacy in my home country.

medical cost 医療費
同義語 medical fee

薬 In Japan, the health insurance covers 70% of the cost. You have to pay 30% of the total cost.

患 I see. But how did you come to that figure? The person before me didn't pay so much.

薬 Your fee depends on your medicines. The fee is calculated based on drug price plus the technical fee for the pharmacist. 4,560 yen is your out-of-pocket fee.

out-of-pocket 自己負担金
関連語 copayment 一部負担金（自己負担金）

患 OK. Then I will pay by debit card.

薬 I'm afraid we don't accept credit or debit cards. We only accept cash.
Would that be all right?

患 I see. Do you have change for 5,000 yen?

薬 Certainly. 440 yen is your change.

5・2　Useful Expressions

■ Let's learn how to describe *symptoms*： skin, urinary and genital organs

(1) I have _____ⒶⒶ_____.

  Ⓐ： a skin rash（湿疹）   warts（いぼ）   acne（にきび）

    sunburn pain（日焼けしたあとが痛い）

    severe athlete's foot（水虫がひどい）

    an itchy eruption on my genitals（陰部に湿疹ができて痒い）

    dry skin all over my body（体中の皮膚がカサカサだ）

    a bruise on my arm（打撲で腕に内出血を起こした）

    frequent urination（頻尿である）

    difficulty urinating and have to strain to start a stream（排尿が困難で
     ひどく力まなければならない）

    a greenish vaginal discharge（緑っぽいおりものがある）

    irregular menstruation（月経の周期が不規則だ）

    vaginal bleeding after my period（月経後に性器出血がある）

    abnormal bleeding（不正出血がある）

(2) My skin is _____Ⓑ_____.

  Ⓑ： very sore（ヒリヒリする）   tingling（ピリピリする）

    very itchy（すごく痒い）

(3) I feel _____Ⓒ_____.

  Ⓒ： itchy（皮膚がとても痒い）

    an itching/burning sensation when urinating（排尿時にしみるように
     痛む）

    a need to pee urgently, but can pass only a few drops（尿意を頻繁に
     感じるのだが，わずかしか尿がでない）

    severe pain during sexual intercourse（性交中に強い痛みを感じる）

(4) I noticed ＿＿＿Ⓓ＿＿＿.

　　Ⓓ: bloody urine/blood in my urine（血尿）

　　　 cloudy urine and it's strong smelling（尿が混濁して悪臭）

(5) I got burnt by boiling water.（熱湯でやけどした）

(6) I was stung by a bee.（蜂に刺された）

Work in Pairs

One partner asks about physical conditions. His/her partner tries to name a few symptoms from (1)–(6) above. Change roles.

Example

Ⓐ What's wrong?

Ⓑ I got burnt by boiling water.

Answers:

Ⓐ ＿＿＿＿＿＿＿＿＿＿＿＿＿＿＿＿＿＿＿＿＿＿

Ⓑ ＿＿＿＿＿＿＿＿＿＿＿＿＿＿＿＿＿＿＿＿＿＿

5・3　Pronunciation Practice

■ Pronounce the following words with special emphasis on accent, rhythm, and stress, etc...　◀)) Track 26

1. itchy
   [ítʃi]

2. rash
   [rǽʃ]

3. acne
   [ǽkni]

4. out-of-pocket
   音節 óut-of-pócket

5. debit
   [débit]

6. debt
   [dét]

7. urine
   [júərin]

8. bruise
   [brúːz]

9. certainly
   [sə́ːrtnli]

5・4　Speak Like a Pharmacist in English

■ Answer the following questions orally in English.

Questions :

1. Tell a patient how much her medications will be in yen.

_____

2. Tell a patient how much Japanese health insurance covers.

_____

3. Tell a patient how drug fees are calculated.

_____

4. Explain to the patient that the pharmacy only accepts cash.

_____

5. Tell the patient how much change she will get.

_____

5・5   Dictation

教)) Track 27   ■ Listen carefully and write down what is said.

Answers :

1. _____

2. _____

3. _____

4. _____

5. _____

6. _____

7. _____

8. _____

5 · 6   Reading Comprehension

■ Read the following passage within 5 minutes and answer all the questions Track 28
orally in English.

If health insurance in Japan is roughly classified, there are three types of health insurance. Social health insurance is coverage provided through an individual's employer, etc. The latter-stage elderly healthcare system is coverage for individuals aged 75 or older. National Health Insurance (hereinafter "NHI") is coverage for individuals not covered by social health insurance. Every person residing in Japan is required to enroll in one of the three types of insurance (compulsory insurance). Foreign nationals residing in Japan are also required to enroll in NHI if they meet certain conditions.

出 典: 京都市, "国民健康保険の手引 (四箇国語パンフレット)" 〔平成 31 年度版 (令和元年度版)〕 より転載.

Questions (Listen to the recording.)　　　　　　　

Answers:

1. _____

2. _____

3. _____

4. _____

5. _____

5 · 7   Listening Comprehension

Track 30   ■ Listen carefully and answer all the questions orally in English.

Questions:

1. In this explanation, where do you live?
2. What is your insurance card proving?
3. How many insurance cards do you have?
4. When is your insurance card necessary?
5. In which medical institutions can you use the card?
6. What percent of medical costs incurred do you pay when you fail to present your insurance card?

Answers:

1. _____

2. _____

3. _____

4. _____

5. _____

6. _____

5 · 8   Make Your Own Dialog

■ Based on what you studied in this unit, work with a partner to make a dialog in English between a pharmacist and a patient.

Situation

Make a dialog where you tell the patient how much their medications will cost. Be ready to explain to her why they cost what they do (with or without Japanese health insurance).

Answers：

A _____

B _____

A _____

B _____

A _____

B _____

A _____

B _____

COLUMN　　　　　テクノロジーが医療にもたらすもの

　私たちはすでにさまざまなテクノロジーに囲まれて生活していますが，医療の世界においても発展や応用にテクノロジーが貢献していることは誰も疑わないと思います．最近ではビッグデータの利活用で医薬品開発のプロセスが大きく変わってきたり，外科手術にロボット"ダヴィンチ（da Vinci）"が導入されたりと，治療の選択肢はテクノロジーによってさらなる広がりをみせています．

　現在，次の一手として期待されているのが人工知能 AI（artificial intelligence）です．AI は医療の根本を変えてしまうかもしれないといわれていますが，それは"診断"において誤診をなくすための切り札と考えられているからです．人間の脳神経回路をモデルにした多層構造アルゴリズムにより，着目すべき特徴や組合わせを AI 自らが考えて決定する"ディープラーニング（深層学習）"を用いた診断は，画像認識といった領域ではすでに人間を凌駕しつつあります．

　一方で，患者の気持ちを理解する医療従事者は必要ですし，医療に挑戦する人間の価値はこれからも変わりません．テクノロジーを道具として正確に認識し，AI によりもたらされる人類の英知を超えた最良の選択を正しく使いこなすことが求められています．　　　　　　　　　　（荒川基記）

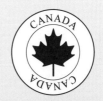

カナダの薬学教育と薬剤師の職域

　"臨床能力を備えた薬剤師の育成を目指して"を掲げて導入された6年制薬学教育も定着し，日本の薬剤師業務は，病院薬剤師は病棟業務へ，薬局薬剤師はかかりつけ薬剤師の業務など，"モノ"から"人"へと大きく変化しました．また，2015年には，新しい薬学教育モデル・コアカリキュラムが施行され，チーム医療への参画や薬物療法についてなど臨床能力を向上させる教育が盛り込まれています．しかし，2年間の臨床薬学教育が追加された6年制薬学部を卒業しても学位は"学士"のままです．カナダでは，患者ケアの高度な教育を受けた学部卒業後には薬学博士（Doctor of Pharmacy: Pharm.D）の称号が与えられています．また，薬剤師に処方権が与えられている州もあります．薬剤師が薬を処方できる…夢のような話ですね．そこで，薬剤師に処方権が与えられているカナダの薬学教育についてご紹介したいと思います．

1. カナダの医療事情

　カナダは，総面積9,984,670 km^{2}の広大な国土をもち，ロッキー山脈やナイアガラの滝など豊かな自然に囲まれた国です．10の州（province）と三つの準州（territory）からなり，人口は3695万と多くありません．薬局数は8870軒，薬剤師数は3万9000人，人口10万人あたりの薬剤師数は95人で，日本の219.6人の半分以下です．

　医療制度は，メディケアとよばれる国民皆保険制度を採用しています．医療費については，患者負担が一切なく，すべてを税財源で公的に負担していますが，眼科，歯科診療，処方薬剤（入院中は無料），リハビリ治療などは全額個人負担になります．

　また，カナダは家庭医（family doctor）が制度化されています．医療機関を利用する場合は，まず地域の家庭医を受診し，専門医への受診は家庭医の紹介が必要となります．しかし，医師は非常に少なく，専門医への受診には数カ月〜1年先まで予約が取れない状況です．日本では3割の負担はありますが，すべての医療サービスが公的保険で賄われ，医療機関へもフリーアクセスで行くことができ，待ち時間も少ない点が魅力といえます．

2. カナダの薬学教育

　現在，カナダには薬学部のある大学が10校あります．なかでもアルバータ州にあるアルバータ州立大学薬学部は歴史が古く，薬学教育プログラムは1914年に医学部として1年間の卒業証明（diploma）と2年間の学位（degree）で始まりました．このプログラムは，1917年から1939年にかけて理学部の理学士号（Bachelor of Science: BSc）となり，1955年に薬学部が設立されました．

　カナダの薬学部は，日本と異なり高校を卒業してから直接薬学部に入学できるわけではありません．まず大学に入学して，1年〜数年で英語，生物学，無機化学，有機化学，数学，統計学の

単位を取得する必要があります．これらの単位を取得後，薬学部に入学する志望理由や将来の夢，仕事に関連した経験，ボランティア経験などに関する小論文とOSCE（objective structured clinical examination）に類似した"態度・資質"が求められます．これらを総合的に評価し条件を満たした学生のみが薬学部への入学を許可されます．大学での講義科目は日本の薬学部と類似していますが，コミュニケーションに焦点を当てたSGD（small group discussion）方式による患者インタビューなどを重視しており，授業内容や方法に大きな相違があります．特徴としては，低学年から現場を経験する実務実習が組込まれていることです．実務実習は，1年生でボランティアのプログラムへの参加と薬局実習，2年生で病院実習など，4年間で4回の実務実習が組込まれており，早い時期から現場を経験する機会を与えています．日本でも1年次に現場を経験する見学型の早期体験実習が取入れられていますが，カナダの場合は見学にとどめずボランティアとして直接患者と接する機会を与えています．

　アルバータ州立大学薬学部は，2018年の秋学期から従来のBSc課程がPharm.D課程に切替わりました．2018年の入学生からは薬学部を卒業するとPharm.Dの学位が取得できます．Pharm.Dとは，患者ケアの高度な教育を提供する学部卒業後に与えられる専門的および職業的な（professional）学位で，研究に焦点を当てた学問的な（academic）Ph.D（Doctor of Philosophy）とは異なります．Pharm.D課程は2年間の薬学部前課程（pre-pharmacy）と4年間の専門課程からなり，専門課程では大学での講義のほかに実際の患者での実習（実地トレーニング）があります．最終学年には地域医療，病院，プライマリーケアネットワークを含む40週間の実習が組込まれています．また，アルバータ州立大学では2017〜2022年度の卒業生と現場の薬剤師にもPharm.Dのプログラムを提供しています．

3．カナダの薬剤師業務

　カナダでは州ごとに法律が異なります．同時に医療制度も異なり，薬剤師に与えられた権限も異なります．次ページの図にカナダの薬剤師会（Canadian Pharmacist Association）が提示した州ごとの薬剤師の職域を示しましたが，カナダで薬剤師が処方権を得ている州はアルバータ州だけです．アルバータ州ではPharm.Dを取得している薬剤師は，病気のスクリーニング，薬物の管理と処方，予防接種の提供に関与することができます．薬物の処方は，麻薬，ベンゾジアゼピン，バルビツール酸，同化ステロイドおよび薬物規制法（Controlled Drugs and Substances Act）で規制されている薬物以外のすべての医療用医薬品（Schedule 1）を処方することができます．他州の薬剤師との大きな違いです．

4．アルバータ州立大学薬学部への留学経験──薬学生へのメッセージ

　日本にクリニカル・ファーマシー（clinical pharmacy）やファーマシューティカル・ケア（pharmaceutical care）という言葉が入ってきた1990年代初め，日本の薬剤師はおもに調剤室の内で薬の調製をすることを業務としていました．1974年には実質的な医薬分業が実施されましたが，1990年代初期の分業率は20％にも達していませんでした．そのころ，北米の薬剤師はすでに病棟で直接患者と関わるクリニカル・ファーマシーの業務をしており，医薬分業率は

		BC	AB	SK	MB	ON	QC	NB	NS	PEI	NL	NWT	YT	NU
処方権（処方薬）規制薬物以外の新しい処方薬治療の開始	すべての処方薬を単独で処方	X	✓	X	X	X	X	X	X	X	X	X	X	X
	共同薬物治療管理業務	X	✓	✓	✓	X	X	X	✓	X	X	X	X	X
	軽度の疾患に対する処方	X	✓	✓	✓	P	✓	✓	✓	✓	X	X	X	X
	禁煙に対する処方	X	✓	✓	✓	✓	✓	✓	✓	✓	✓	X	X	X
	緊急時の処方	✓	✓	✓	✓	✓	X	X	✓	✓	✓	X	X	X
医師の許可なく処方を変更する	すべての処方薬を単独で変更	X	✓	X	X	X	X	X	X	X	X	X	X	X
	規制薬以外の処方薬を単独で変更	X	✓	X	✓	✓	✓	✓	✓	✓	✓	X	X	X
	代替薬への変更	✓	✓	✓	✓	X	P	✓	✓	✓	✓	X	P	X
	用量，剤形，レジメンの変更	✓	✓	✓	✓	✓	✓	✓	✓	✓	✓	X	✓	X
	治療継続のための処方更新/延長	✓	✓	✓	✓	✓	✓	✓	✓	✓	✓	X	P	X
注射の権限（皮下および筋肉注射）	すべての薬剤およびワクチン	P	✓	✓	✓	P	X	P	✓	✓	✓	X	X	X
	ワクチン	✓	✓	✓	✓	✓	X	✓	✓	✓	✓	X	X	X
	インフルエンザワクチン	✓	✓	✓	✓	✓	✓	✓	✓	✓	✓	X	X	X
臨床検査	臨床検査のオーダーと判読	X	✓	P	✓	X	✓	P	P	✓	✓	X	X	X
テクニシャン		✓	✓	✓	✓	✓	X	✓	✓	✓	✓	X	X	X

✓: 管轄区域で実施　　X: 実施されていない　　P: 実施については未定
BC: ブリティッシュコロンビア，AB: アルバータ，SK: サスカチュワン，MB: マニトバ，ON: オンタリオ，QC: ケベック，NB: ニューブランズウィック，NS: ノバスコシア，PEI: プリンスエドワードアイランド，NL: ニューファンドランド・ラブラドール，NWT: ノースウエスト準州，YT: ユーコン準州，NU: ヌナブト準州

図　カナダにおける州ごとの薬剤師の職域（Canadian Pharmacist Association による）

ほぼ100％でした．そんな北米の薬剤師の業務を見てみたいという衝動にかられ，1997年に母校の東邦大学から姉妹校のアルバータ州立大学薬学部に留学しました．アルバータ州立大学薬学部では，おもに専門課程の講座を受講しました．専門課程ではすでに薬物療法を重視した教育をしており，実習では患者の薬物療法の問題点（drug related problem；DRP）を抽出して，グループで討論する（small group discussion；SGD）という授業方式を取入れていました．日本の大学でも今では当たり前のようにSGDを取入れた授業をしていますが，当時はこの画期的な授業手法や薬物療法（therapeutics），抗微生物学（antimicrobial）の講義に目から鱗が落ちるような思いでした．

また，クラスメートたちのモチベーションの高さや医療にかける想いには目を見張るものがあり，深い感銘を受けました．現在のアルバータ州立大学でのPharm.D課程の設立や処方権の獲得は，薬学教育への開拓と医療にかける熱い想いで長い年月をかけて築きあげられたものではないでしょうか．

近年，海外に留学する日本人が減っているといわれています．特に薬学部では，6年制になってから海外へ目を向ける学生が少なくなっているように思われます．筆者は，カナダでの留学生活を通してかけがえのないものを得ることができました．薬学生が在学中に長期の留学をすることは，現状では難しいでしょう．しかし，幸いなことに，現在ではどこの薬系大学でも短期の海外研修プログラムがあります．短期の海外研修に参加して異文化にふれることが海外へ目を向けるきっかけとなるはずです．卒業後，一人でも多くの学生に留学への道を歩んでほしいと思います．

（渡辺朋子）

PART Ⅱ

Drugstore

UNIT 6

Category 1 OTC Drug Sales

処方箋なしで購入できる医薬品は，"一般用医薬品（OTC医薬品）"と"要指導医薬品"に大別される．さらに，一般用医薬品にはリスクに応じた三つの区分があり，医薬品のリスクレベルに応じて，第一類医薬品，第二類医薬品および第三類医薬品に分類され，それぞれ販売時の陳列や薬剤師などの専門家の関わり方，情報提供の仕方が定められている．

リスクが最も低い第三類医薬品および第二類医薬品は，資格認定試験を受けた登録販売者でも販売が可能である．特に第三類医薬品では情報提供も義務付けられていない．しかしながら，第一類医薬品の販売は薬剤師に限定され，販売時には書面による情報提供が義務付けられているため，薬剤師がいなければ販売することができない．

Category 1

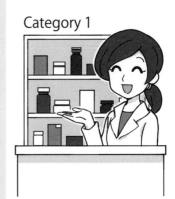

6・1 Dialog

■ Listen to the dialog and memorize it.

 Track 31

登 Hi, what are you looking for?

客 I have had joint pain since I had a fall last week.

登 Do you have any other problems?

客 I also have lower back pain. Do you have some Loxonin S?

登 Yes, we do. Loxonin S is classified as a first category medicine. If you would like to buy it, by law, a pharmacist needs to explain how to take it. Do you have time?

客 OK, but please hurry.

薬 Thank you for waiting. My name is Ishida. I am a pharmacist here. I heard you have had joint pain and lower back pain for a week, and you would like to buy Loxonin S. Is that right?

客 Yes.

登: 登録販売者

joint pain 関節痛

lower back pain
腰痛

薬 How are you feeling right now?

客 My joints and lower back still hurt.

薬 What kind of pain is it?

dull pain 鈍痛

severe pain 激痛

客 It is dull pain. But when I walk, I have severe pain. Will Loxonin S relieve my pain?

薬 Loxonin S will help relieve your joint and lower back pain. Loxonin S is categorized as a high risk drug, if you would like to buy this, I need to explain about the medication to you. Is that all right for you?

客 Sure.

薬 OK, please have a seat.

6・2 Useful Expressions

■ Let's learn how to describe *symptoms*: respiratory and digestive system, injury

(1) I have _____Ⓐ_____.

Ⓐ: heartburn/a sour stomach（胸焼け）　　anorexia（食欲不振）
　　shortness of breath（息切れ）　　　　a rapid heartbeat（動悸）
　　trouble breathing（呼吸困難）　　　　a migraine（片頭痛）
　　severe muscle aches（ひどい筋肉痛）
　　bad insomnia（ひどく眠れない / ひどい不眠症）
　　blood in my stool（便に血が混じっている）

(2) I am numb in my leg./I have a numb leg.（脚の感覚がない）

(3) I sprained my ankle/finger.（足をくじいた / つき指をした）

(4) I got bit by a dog.（犬に噛まれた）

Work in Pairs

One partner asks about physical conditions. His/her partner tries to name a few symptoms from (1)-(4) above. Change roles.

Example
Ⓐ What's wrong?
Ⓑ I sprained my ankle.

Answers:

A _____

B _____

6·3   Pronunciation Practice

■ Pronounce the following words with special emphasis on accent, rhythm, ◀))) Track 32
and stress, etc...

1. insomnia
   [insámniə]

2. numb
   [nʌ́m]

3. joint pain
   [dʒɔ́int péin]

4. back pain
   [bǽk péin]

5. ankle
   [ǽŋkl]

6. diabetes
   [dáiəbíːtis -tiːz]

7. respiratory
   [réspərətɔ̀ːri]

8. migraine
   [máigrein]

9. sprain
   [spréin]

6·4   Speak Like a Pharmacist in English

■ Answer the following questions orally in English.

Questions:

1. How do you start communication with a customer?

   _____

2. How do you ask a customer about his symptoms?

   _____

3. Ask the customer if he has ever had this illness before.

   _____

4. Ask the customer if he has any allergies.

   _____

5. Ask the customer if he is taking any other medicines.

   _____

6・5   Dictation

 ■ Listen carefully and write down what is said.

Answers:

1. _____

2. _____

3. _____

4. _____

5. _____

6. _____

7. _____

8. _____

6・6   Reading Comprehension

 ■ Read the following passage within 5 minutes and answer all the questions orally in English.

Acetaminophen is a safe and effective pain reliever that benefits millions of consumers. However, taking too much could lead to serious liver damage. There are about 600 products that contain acetaminophen, including cough and cold products and sleep aids. It is also an ingredient in many prescription pain relievers. The Food and Drug Administration warns consumers that all over-the-counter pain relievers should be taken with care to avoid serious problems that can occur with misuse.

Parents should be cautious when giving acetaminophen to children. For example, the infant drop formula is three times stronger than the children's suspension. To help make sure your infant is getting the infants' formula and your child is getting the children's formula, you should read and follow the directions on the label every time you use a medicine. Parents are cautioned against giving any acetaminophen or cough and cold medications to children under 2 years of age without the advice of a health care provider.

出 典: *Health Bulletin*: *Use Caution with Pain Relievers* (*acetaminophen*), U.S. FDA の ウエブサイト〔https://www.fda.gov/drugs/safe-use-over-counter-pain-relievers-and-fever-reducers/health-bulletin-use-caution-pain-relievers-acetaminophen（2019 年 11 月 現 在 ）〕 より転載.

Questions（Listen to the recording.）

Answers：

1. _____

2. _____

3. _____

4. _____

5. _____

6. _____

6・7 Listening Comprehension

■ Listen carefully and answer all the questions orally in English.

Questions：

1. What is important to avoid overdosing by mistake?

2. What is important when you take acetaminophen?

3. What functions of the liver are mentioned?

4. What makes your liver unable to process acetaminophen safely?

5. When does your body produce more of the toxic chemical?

6. What could happen when more of the toxic chemical remains in your body?

Answers：

1. _____

2. _____

3. _____

4. _____

5. _____

6. _____

6・8   Make Your Own Dialog

■ Based on what you studied in this unit, work with a partner to make a dialog in English between a pharmacist and a patient.

Situation

Mr. Smith came to your drugstore to get some pain-reliever. Ask him as many questions as you can to choose the most appropriate medicine for him.

Answers：

A _____

B _____

A _____

B _____

A

B

A

B

医療費の高騰とセルフメディケーション

　日本人にとって，医療費を保険でカバーされることは当たり前であるが，この国民皆保険とよばれる制度は，世界でも類をみない優良な制度である．しかし，この制度は働き手が保険料を納めることにより成り立つ制度のため，少子高齢化が進む日本では医療費の高騰がさらに進み，このままではやがて国民皆保険制度自体が崩壊する恐れがある．

　国民皆保険制度を守るために医療費の削減を目指した数々の対策がなされているが，その一つにセルフメディケーションの推進がある．セルフメディケーションとは，"自分自身の健康に責任をもち，軽度な身体の不調は自分で手当てすること"（WHOの定義）であり，軽度な疾病やけがの場合に，直接ドラッグストアなどでOTC医薬品を購入し，自ら治療することもセルフメディケーションの一環である．セルフメディケーションを行うことで病院の受診料などの医療費を減らし，結果的に医療費削減が期待される．

　OTC医薬品による治療では，薬剤師は唯一患者に関わる医療従事者であるため，大きな責任を担うとともに活躍が期待されている．

（中島理恵）

UNIT 7

Doping

ドーピングとは，トレーニングやスポーツにおいて，アスリートが禁止されている物質や方法によって競技能力を高め，意図的に自分だけが優位に立ち，勝利を得ようとする行為のことである．禁止物質を意図的に使用することだけでなく，意図的かどうかに関わらず，ルールに反するさまざまな競技能力を高める方法や，それらの行為を隠すことも含めて，ドーピングとよぶ．

禁止物質として，はじめに思い浮かぶのはステロイドであるが，他にも興奮剤，ホルモン，利尿薬，麻薬およびマリファナなどがある．医薬品には，禁止薬物が含まれていることが多く，アスリートに医薬品を提供する場合には，禁止物質の有無を確認する必要がある．漢方薬にも麻黄*などの禁止物質が含まれていることがあるため注意が必要である．特に OTC 医薬品を販売するときには注意を要する．（＊ 禁止物質のエフェドリンが含有されている．）

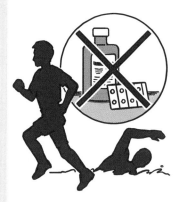

7・1　Dialog

 Track 37　■ Listen to the dialog and memorize it.

薬 Good morning! What brings you here today?

the chills 寒気

客 I have the chills. I think I caught a cold.

cold かぜ

薬 Do you have a fever or a cough?

sore throat 咽喉炎,
咽頭痛

客 I don't have a fever, but I have a cough and sore throat. Do you have any medicines that will work for these symptoms?

薬 I see. I recommend this medicine.

客 Is this a Kampo medicine? I would like some Kampo cold medicine.

薬 No, this is not. Why do you think Kampo medicines are for you?

客 I am worried about a doping test because I will be in the national athletics meet starting the day after tomorrow. I heard Kampo medicines don't have any prohibited doping substances.

薬 While there can be prohibited substances in effective Kampo cold medicines, this is not a Kampo medicine, so it won't be a problem.

客 I see. I will take this. Thank you very much.

prohibited
substance
禁止物質
同義語 prohibited
component

7・2   Useful Expressions

■ Let's learn how to describe *dosage forms and usage*：

① Oral medicine/internal remedy（内服薬）

(1) I take/have/get ＿＿＿Ⓐ＿＿＿.

Ⓐ： a powder（散剤）   tablets（錠剤）   granules（顆粒剤）

capsules（カプセル剤）   a pill（丸薬）   emulsions（液剤）

a liquid dosage form（液状製剤）   oral suspensions（懸濁剤）

an elixir（エリキシル剤）   a syrup（シロップ剤）

troches/lozenges（トローチ剤）   sublingual tablets（舌下錠）

(2) Please ＿＿＿Ⓑ＿＿＿.

Ⓑ： suck it（なめる）   don't chew/crush it（かみ砕かない）

swallow it（丸のみする）with a glass of water/without chewing

don't swallow it（まる飲みしない）

let it dissolve under your tongue（舌の下において溶かす）

place it in your mouth and allow it to dissolve slowly

shake（振る）it well just before you measure a dose and take it with
a full glass of water

don't break or crush tablets, or open capsules without following the
instructions（自分勝手に錠剤を割ったり，つぶしたり，カプセルの
中身を取出してはいけない）

Work in Pairs

One partner asks how to take or use a medicine from (1) above. His/
her partner tries to explain the usage from (2) above. Change roles.

Example

Ⓐ How can I take these tablets?

Ⓑ Please swallow them with a glass of water.

Answers：

A
_____

B
_____

7・3   Pronunciation Practice

🔊)) Track 38   ■ Pronounce the following words with special emphasis on accent, rhythm, and stress, etc...

1. capsule
   [kǽpsəl]

2. dosage
   [dóusidʒ]

3. dose
   [dóus]

4. granule
   [grǽnjuːl]

5. adverse reaction
   [ædvə́ːrs riǽkʃən]

6. pancreas
   [pǽnkriəs]

7. incubator
   [íŋkjubèitər]

8. inhibitor
   [inhíbitər]

9. lozenge
   [lázindʒ]

7・4   Speak Like a Pharmacist in English

■ Answer the following questions orally in English.

Questions：

1. Ask the patient about her symptoms.

   _____

2. Tell the patient what medicine you recommend.

   _____

3. Explain how to take a pain reliever.

   _____

4. Ask the patient about her pain.

   _____

5. Explain a Kampo medicine.

   _____

7·5 Dictation

■ Listen carefully and write down what is said.   教))) Track 39

Answers:

1. _____

2. _____

3. _____

4. _____

5. _____

6. _____

7. _____

8. _____

7·6 Reading Comprehension

■ Read the following passage within 5 minutes and answer all the questions))) Track 40
orally in English.

It's easy to grab the first cold and flu medication on the shelf, but as an athlete you need to be extra cautious in checking if any medication or other substance you are taking is prohibited in- or out-of-competition.

You should also be aware that supplements and herbal products can contain prohibited substances. Supplements and herbal products are not regulated in the same way as medicines, so they can contain substances not listed on the label, and are at greater risk from cross-contamination from other substances manufactured on the same equipment.

So remember, before you take a medication or other substance to get over your cold or flu always check your substances on Global DRO (The Global Drug Reference Online) for its status in sport.

出 典: *Blog*: *Don't let a cold take you out of action for four years...*, Australian Sports Anti-Doping Authority のウエブサイト〔https://www.asada.gov.au/news/blog-dont-let-cold-take-you-out-action-four-years（2019 年 11 月現在)〕より転載.

 Questions（Listen to the recording.）

Answers：

1. _____

2. _____

3. _____

4. _____

5. _____

7・7   Listening Comprehension

 Track 42   ■ Listen carefully and answer all the questions orally in English.

Questions：

1. How many ways are there to obtain medicine?

2. When do you need to remind your doctor that you are an athlete and are subject to anti-doping regulations?

3. If your doctor is unsure about your medication, who should you consult?

4. Who can you consult when you need to take an over-the-counter medication?

5. If a pharmacist is not available, who else can help you with your OTC meds?

Answers：

1. _____

2. _____

3. _____

4. _____

5. _____

7・8　Make Your Own Dialog

■ Based on what you studied in this unit, work with a partner to make a dialog in English between a pharmacist and a patient.

Situation

Make a dialog where you counsel a patient on which medicine to take for a cold. You may or may not recommend a Kampo medicine.

Answers：

A _____

B _____

A _____

B _____

A _____

B _____

A _____

B _____

COLUMN　　　　　　　　コンパニオン診断薬と分子標的医薬品

　コンパニオン診断（companion diagnostics；CoDx）は，使用する治療薬に最も奏効すると予測される患者を選択し，その患者に対して最適な治療を行うための検査です．CoDx は，バイオマーカーあるいは薬剤の標的分子を対象とし，有効な患者を選択するための診断方法として用いられ，通常の臨床検査とは区別されています．

　薬物療法に際して用いられる体外診断薬で，特定の医薬品の有効性や安全性を一層高めるために，その使用対象者に該当するかどうかをあらかじめ検査する目的で使用される診断薬はコンパニオン診断薬といわれています．したがって，新規の検査であれば医薬品と対になって開発・承認されることが重要になります．コンパニオン診断薬は，個別化医療の一端を担うものとして注目されており，たとえば悪性腫瘍などに対する標準的な薬物療法を施行するうえで必要なものとなっています．一方で，医薬品のバイオマーカーに対して承認された CoDx が必ずしも存在しないことや診療報酬上の課題により新規の CoDx の導入が問題となることがあります．　　　　　（日髙慎二）

UNIT 8

Recommending an OTC Drug

OTC とは，over-the-counter の略で，カウンター越しに薬を販売するかたちに由来する．正式には，一般用医薬品といい，薬局やドラッグストアで，医師からの処方箋なしに自らの判断で簡単に購入できる．自分自身で軽度な体調不良の治療や健康上の問題を予防することに役立つ身近な薬であり，一般的に安全な薬と考えられている．しかし，ときに有害事象などの不快な症状をひき起こすことがある．

OTC 医薬品の販売に関わる専門家は，消費者が OTC 医薬品を安全で効果的に使用するために，消費者が OTC 医薬品を選択する際に適切なアドバイスを行い，販売する薬に対する情報提供と服薬指導を行う義務がある．安全かつ効果的な OTC 医薬品の提供も薬剤師の重要な役割である．

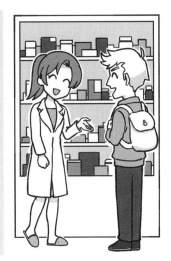

8・1 　Dialog

■ Listen to the dialog and memorize it.

🔊)) Track 43

薬 Is there anything I can help you with?

客 I would like some Bufferin.

薬 What seems to be troubling you?

客 I have a slight fever and a runny nose. It seems like I have a cold.

薬 Hmm...Bufferin won't help a runny nose.

runny nose 鼻水
同義語 running nose

客 I see. Which medicine will work on these symptoms? Which medicine do you recommend for me?

薬 Have you ever had any adverse reactions to medicine before?

客 No, I haven't.

薬 OK. I recommend this medicine.

客 This medicine won't make me drowsy, right?

drowsy 眠い
同義語 drowsiness

薬 I am afraid not. This medicine may make you drowsy. Do not drive a car or operate machinery while you are taking this medicine. Otherwise I recommend a Kampo medicine. Kampo medicines won't make you drowsy. But this medicine works better than a Kampo medicine.

客 OK. Then I will take this medicine.

薬 Do you have any questions?

客 For now, no.

薬 Please contact us if you have any unusual problems while taking this medicine.

8・2　Useful Expressions

■ Let's learn how to describe *dosage forms and usage*：

External medicines/topical agents（外用薬）

(1) I use ＿＿＿ Ⓐ ＿＿＿.

Ⓐ： inhalations/inhalants（吸入剤）   inhalers（吸入器）
    aerosols（エアゾル剤）   anal suppositories（坐剤）
    vaginal suppositories（膣坐剤）   an ointment（軟膏剤）
    gargles（含嗽剤）   enemas（浣腸剤）
    eye drops（点眼剤）   nose drops（点鼻剤）
    ear drops（点耳剤）   a cream（クリーム）
    a lotion（ローション / 水薬）   a gel（ゲル剤）
    medicated patches（貼り薬）   tapes/poultices（貼付剤）
    a cold/hot compress（冷・温湿布薬）

(2) Please ＿＿＿ Ⓑ ＿＿＿.

Ⓑ： apply/put it on（塗る / 付ける）   rub it（擦り込む）
    put/apply/place it（貼る / 当てる）
    use these eye drops when your eyes are dry（目が乾いたときにさす）
    place one drop into the eye/the ear canal（目 / 外耳道に 1 滴さす）
    insert it deeply into your anus, with the pointed end inserted first
    　　　（尖っている方から肛門内にできるだけ深く入れてください）

Work in Pairs

One partner asks how to take or use a medicine from (1) on page 60. His/her partner tries to explain the usage from (2) on page 60. Change roles.

Example

A How can I take this ointment?

B Apply it to the itchy area. Don't use too much.

Answers:

A _____

B _____

8 · 3   Pronunciation Practice

■ Pronounce the following words with special emphasis on accent, rhythm, and stress, etc...   ◀)) Track 44

1. Bufferin
    [bʌ́fərin]

2. acetaminophen
    [əsìːtəmínəfən]

3. inhalant
    [inhéilənt]

4. ointment
    [ɔ́intmənt]

5. ibuprofen
    [àibjuːpróufən]

6. suppository
    [səpázətɔ̀ːri]

7. laboratory
    [lǽbərətɔ̀ːri]

8. supplement
    [sʌ́pləmənt]

9. gargle
    [ɡáːrɡl]

8 · 4   Speak Like a Pharmacist in English

■ Answer the following questions orally in English.

Questions:

1. A patient is looking for something in your drugstore, what should you say?

_____

2. Ask if the patient has had any adverse reactions to a medicine before.

_____

3. Tell the patient a precaution about a medicine.

_____

4. Ask the patient if he has any questions.

_____

5. What would you say to a customer who has an adverse reaction after taking a medicine?

_____

8 · 5   Dictation

 ■ Listen carefully and write down what is said.

Answers：

1. _____

2. _____

3. _____

4. _____

5. _____

6. _____

7. _____

8. _____

8 · 6   Reading Comprehension

 ■ Read the following passage within 5 minutes and answer all the questions orally in English.

We tend to think of over-the-counter (OTC) painkillers as perfectly safe. If you can buy a drug sitting next to the toothpaste and shampoo, how dangerous could it be?

But even these drugs do have risks. And if you have an ulcer, you need to be very careful before popping over-the-counter painkillers. Many commonplace drugs—such as aspirin, ibuprofen, and naproxen... can irritate the stomach lining, aggravating ulcers and potentially causing serious problems.

"People think that if a medicine is available over-the-counter, it has no risks," says Byron Cryer, MD, a spokesman for the American Gastroenterological Association. "But about a third of all ulcers are caused by aspirin and other painkillers. More than half of all bleeding ulcers are caused by these drugs."

In fact, according to the American Gastroenterological Association, 103,000 people are hospitalized every year because of side effects from common painkillers. Some 16,500 people die.

出　典：R. Morgan Griffin, *Everyday Pain Relief: Ulcers*, WebMD のウエブサイト〔https://www.webmd.com/digestive-disorders/features/everyday-pain-relief-ulcers#1 （2019 年 11 月現在）〕より転載.

Questions（Listen to the recording.）

Answers：

1. _____

2. _____

3. _____

4. _____

5. _____

6. _____

8·7　Listening Comprehension

🔊)) Track 48　　■ Listen carefully and answer all the questions orally in English.

Questions:

1. What can lower your risk of experiencing gastric pain symptoms?
2. How many ways are mentioned to change your lifestyle?
3. How many times are recommended for having meals a day?
4. What are features of irritating foods?
5. What kinds of adverse effects could be caused by excessive amounts of alcohol?
6. What kinds of ways are there for managing your stress?

Answers:

1. _____

2. _____

3. _____

4. _____

5. _____

6. _____

8·8　Make Your Own Dialog

■ Based on what you studied in this unit, work with a partner to make a dialog in English between a pharmacist and a patient.

Situation

A patient wants a cold medicine that won't make him drowsy. Make a dialog where you recommend a medicine because it doesn't have that side effect.

Answers：

A _____

B _____

A _____

B _____

A _____

B _____

A _____

B _____

COLUMN　　　　　　　　**薬の選択と推奨（胃薬）**

　病院で処方される医療用医薬品で使用されている成分のなかには，処方箋なしでOTC医薬品として買えるものがあります．病院に行く時間がない，病院にかかるほどではないような胃の症状があった場合を例に考えます．胃痛や胃潰瘍は，攻撃因子である胃酸と，防御因子である胃粘液・胃粘膜のバランスが崩れ，胃粘膜が胃酸の刺激を受けることによって起こります．NSAIDs（非ステロイド性消炎鎮痛薬），ピロリ菌感染，ストレス，疲労，食生活，喫煙などがバランスを崩す要因です．症状を抑えるには，攻撃因子である胃酸の分泌を減らす，胃酸を中和する，または防御因子の

胃粘膜を保護するなど，攻撃因子と防御因子のバランスを修正する必要があります．

　OTC医薬品の胃腸薬には，胃酸の分泌を抑えるヒスタミン（H_2）受容体拮抗薬，ムスカリン（M_1）受容体拮抗薬のほか，胃酸を中和する制酸薬，荒れた胃粘膜を保護する胃粘膜保護薬，胃の痙攣を抑える鎮痛鎮痙薬などがあります．薬局やドラッグストアの薬剤師や登録販売者に相談して，用法用量，副作用に注意しながら，症状に合った胃薬を選択するとよいでしょう．

　　　　　　　　　　　　　　　　　　（花岡峻輔）

UNIT 9

Medicines Not for Sale as OTC in Japan

医薬品は，処方箋薬（医療用医薬品）と非処方箋薬（一般用医薬品）の二つに大別され，処方箋薬は医師の処方による医薬品であるという点で日本と諸外国は同様である．一方で，非処方箋薬（一般用医薬品）については，各国で販売規制が異なる．すなわち，販売可能な店舗，販売者，承認薬の種類に相違がある．たとえば，米国では，モーニング・アフター・ピル（緊急避妊薬）や胃薬のネキシウム（PPI: proton pump inhibitor）は処方箋なしに薬局やドラッグストアで購入することが可能であるが，これらの医薬品は，日本ではまだ一般用医薬品として承認されていない．したがって，外国人が，一般用医薬品として承認されていない医薬品の購入を求めた場合には，代替薬を推奨するか，医師への受診を促す必要がある．

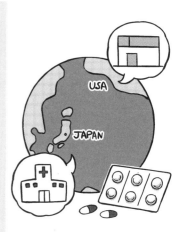

9・1　Dialog

 Track 49　■ Listen to the dialog and memorize it.

heartburn 胸焼け

stomach discomfort 胃部不快感

nausea 吐き気

＊ Nexium（商品名）：一般名は esomeprazole magnesium hydrate.

薬 How can I be of help? What seems to be the problem?

客 I have had heartburn, stomach discomfort, and nausea since last night.

薬 Did you have these complaints after eating a meal?

客 Yes, I did. Do you have Nexium*? My doctor told me that if those symptoms occur, I should take Nexium.

薬 I see. If you would like to take Nexium, you have to see a doctor.

客 Why? I can always buy Nexium at a drug store without a prescription in my home country.

薬 I see. However, Nexium has not been approved as an OTC medicine in Japan.

客 OK. I am traveling and I don't have health insurance. Do you have any medicine that works like Nexium?

薬 We have Gaster 10. Gaster 10 helps prevent stomach acid and relieve your symptoms.

客 OK. I will try Gaster 10.

薬 Please take one tablet when you have heartburn or stomach discomfort. If you still feel heartburn or stomach discomfort after eight hours, take one more tablet. If your symptoms last longer than three days, stop taking this medication and please see a doctor.

客 I understand. Thank you.

薬 Please take care.

9・2　Useful Expressions

■ Let's learn how to describe *dose method*:

(1) Take/have ＿＿＿＿Ⓐ＿＿＿＿.

Ⓐ: one pack once a day/once daily（1日1回，1包ずつ）

two capsules twice a day/two times daily after breakfast and dinner
（1日2回，朝夕食後に2カプセルずつ）

one tablet in the morning and evening（朝と夕に1錠ずつ）

one division on this scale three times a day before meals
（1日3回，毎食前にこの線の1目盛り）

one tablet four times a day, every six hours
（1日4回，6時間ごと1錠ずつ）

one pack three times a day between meals
（1日3回，食間に1包ずつ）

these tablets within thirty minutes after each meal（毎食後30分以内）

these tablets before you go to bed（寝る前にこれらの錠剤を）

one tablet at bedtime（就寝時に1錠）

one capsule on an empty stomach 1 hour before or 2 to 3 hours after
a meal（1カプセル，食前1時間または食後2～3時間の空腹時に）

before breakfast（朝食前）　　these tablets every other day（隔日）

(2) Use/take this medicine when you have ＿＿＿Ⓑ＿＿＿.

Ⓑ: a cough　　pain　　a fever　　a palpitation（動悸がする）

(3) Use/take this medicine when the pain _____Ⓒ_____.

    Ⓒ: persists（持続するとき）   is unbearable（我慢できないとき）

(4) Use/take/apply this medicine _____Ⓓ_____.

    Ⓓ: when you feel dizzy

        when it itches（痒いとき）

        when necessary（必要時，頓服）

        as directed by the doctor（医師の指示どおり）

        with food or milk（食物やミルクと一緒に）

(5) Don't _____Ⓔ_____when you take this medicine.

    Ⓔ: drink alcohol   drive a car

(6) If you haven't eaten, you should not take this medicine.

(7) If you miss a dose of this medicine and become aware of that during a meal, you should take it immediately. However, if you become aware of that after a meal, you should skip the missed dose.

Work in Pairs

One partner asks how to take or use a medicine. His/her partner tries to explain the usage from (1)–(5) above. Change roles.

Example

🅐 How often should I take this?

🅑 Please take it three times a day after meals.

Answers：

🅐 _____

🅑 _____

9・3   Pronunciation Practice

 Track 50   ■ Pronounce the following words with special emphasis on accent, rhythm, and stress, etc...

1. gaster
   [gǽstər]

2. heartburn
   [hártbərn]

3. occur
   [əkə́ːr]

4. diagnose
   [dàiəgnòus, -nòuz]

5. ethyl
   [éθəl]

6. pregnant
   [prégnənt]

7. narcotic
   [nɑːrkátik]

8. cocaine
   [koukéin]

9. marijuana
   [mæ̀rəhwáːnə]

9・4   Speak Like a Pharmacist in English

■ Answer the following questions orally in English.

Questions：

1. Ask a patient when her symptoms started.

   _____

2. Ask a patient how long he has had his symptoms.

   _____

3. Explain to the patient that an OTC medicine outside Japan is a prescription medicine here.

   _____

4. Recommend an alternative medicine to a customer.

   _____

5. How should you always end a conversation with an ill customer or patient?

   _____

9・5   Dictation

■ Listen carefully and write down what is said.   教)) Track 51

Answers：

1. _____

2. _____

3. _____

4. _____

5. _____

6. _____

7. _____

8. _____

9 · 6 Reading Comprehension

Track 52 ■ Read the following passage within 5 minutes and answer all the questions orally in English.

Japanese physicians can often prescribe similar, but not identical, substitutes to medicines available in the U.S. A list of English-speaking medical facilities throughout Japan is available elsewhere on our web site. A Japanese doctor, consulted by phone in advance, is also a good source of information on medications available and/or permitted in Japan.

Some popular medications legal in the U.S., such as Prozac and Viagra, are sold illegally in Japan on the black market. You are subject to arrest and imprisonment if you purchase such drugs illegally while in Japan.

Persons traveling to Japan carrying prescription and non-prescription medications should consult the Japanese Embassy, or a Japanese Consulate, in the United States before leaving the U.S. to confirm whether they will be allowed to bring the particular medication into Japan. A full listing of phone numbers and email addresses is available at http://www.us.emb-japan.go.jp/jicc/consulate-guide.html.

出 典：*Importing or Bringing Medication into Japan for Personal Use*, U.S. Embassy & Consulates in Japan のウエブサイト〔https://jp.usembassy.gov/u-s-citizen-services/doctors/importing-medication/（2019 年 11 月現在）〕より転載.

Questions (Listen to the recording.)

 Track 53

Answers：

1. _____

2. _____

3. _____

4. _____

5. _____

6. _____

9・7 Listening Comprehension

■ Listen carefully and answer all the questions orally in English.

 Track 54

Questions：

1. Give three examples of drugs that cannot be brought into Japan.
2. What is Adderall an example of ?
3. Are OTC medicines from America always OK to bring into Japan?
4. What are two kinds of stimulant drugs you can never bring into Japan—even with a prescription?
5. How much of a legal prescription drug is someone allowed to bring into Japan?
6. What should a visitor from abroad also bring with their prescription medication when visiting Japan?

Answers：

1. _____

2. _____

3. _____

4. _____

5. _____

6. _____

9・8   Make Your Own Dialog

■ Based on what you studied in this unit, work with a partner to make a dialog in English between a pharmacist and a patient.

Situation

Make a dialog where the patient is requesting a medicine after drinking and eating too much. Make sure the medicine is an OTC.

Answers：

A _____

B _____

A _____

B _____

A _____

B _____

A _____

B _____

COLUMN　　リフレーミングを知っていますか？

　私たちはすべての物事を，その人独自の視点で見ています．この物事を見る視点のことを“フレーム”といいます．そして，このフレームを変えることを“リフレーミング”といいます．リフレーミングを行うと，同じ物事であっても，それらの意味が変化し，気分や感情を変えることができます．

　たとえば，仕事で失敗したときに“自分はダメだ”と見るか，“次のために良い経験をした”と見るかで，感じ方が変わります．心理療法や，学校の授業，保健指導などでも活用されていますが，薬剤師が患者の薬物療法を支援する際にも大変有効なスキルです．私たちが出会う出来事に本来は良いも悪いもありません．ただ，それに対して，どう見るか，どう意味づけするかで良いのか悪いのかを決めていて，前向きな気持ちになったり，あるいは嫌な気分を味わってしまったりしているのです．

　もしあなたがリフレーミングを日常的に使えるようになると，こころの状態が一瞬にして変わり，あなたの本来の目的に向かって行動しやすくなります．一つの出来事をいろいろな角度から見るクセをつけておきましょう．そして将来，薬剤師として患者を支援する際にも役立てていきましょう．

（安部　恵）

UNIT 10 Physician Recommendation

OTC 医薬品は，薬局やドラッグストアで医師からの処方箋なしに自らの意思で手軽に購入でき，軽度な身体の不調を自分自身で改善し，健康を維持するのに役立つ便利な医薬品である．しかしながら，消費者はときに的確な自己診断ができないことがある．たとえば，頭痛がまれに脳梗塞や脳出血，脳腫瘍の警告となっていることがある．また，重度の胸焼けは心臓発作の前触れとなっていることがあり，医薬品を適切に使用するためには，医学的な知識を必要とする．薬剤師は，消費者が OTC 医薬品の購入を求めたときには，薬学的な観点で購入者の状態を判断し，購入者がかかえる問題が OTC 医薬品の使用で改善できないと判断した場合には，速やかに医師への診断を促す必要がある．

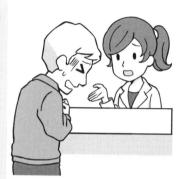

10・1　Dialog

 Track 55　■ Listen to the dialog and memorize it.

headache 頭痛

客 Excuse me, do you have any good medicine for a headache?

薬 What's the matter? You look pale.

客 I have had a headache for the past few days.

薬 Do you have any other symptoms?

stiff shoulder
肩こり

客 I have had stiff shoulders.

vomiting 嘔吐

薬 Do you have nausea or feel like vomiting?

客 Yes, I am suffering from nausea today.

薬 Have you been taking any medications?

客 I have been taking a pain killer from a drug store, but it doesn't seem to work.

blood pressure
血圧

薬 OK. Do you have abnormally high blood pressure?

客 Yes, I do.

薬 I see. In that case, OTC drugs may not be appropriate. You need to see a doctor.

客 OK. Could you introduce me to a good physician near here?

薬 I recommend Dr. Oka. He speaks English. His clinic is in the next building. I can make an appointment for you.

客 That will help me greatly.

10・2 Useful Expressions

■ Let's learn how to describe *drug efficacy and side effects*： popular medicines

(1) This is/these are ＿＿＿＿Ⓐ＿＿＿＿.

 Ⓐ： an antipyretic/a fever reducer（解熱薬）
  analgesics/a pain killer/pain relievers（鎮痛薬）
  anorexics/appetite suppressants/diet pills（食欲抑制薬）
  anticoagulants/blood thinners（抗凝血薬）
  antihistamines/cold and allergy medicines（抗ヒスタミン薬）
  antihyperlipidemics/cholesterol reducers（高脂血症治療薬）
  antihypertensives/high blood pressure reducers（降圧薬）
  hypnotics/sleeping pills（睡眠薬）
  laxatives/stool softeners（緩下薬）
  tranquilizers/nerve pills（精神安定剤）

(2) They are medicines that ＿＿＿＿Ⓑ＿＿＿＿.

 Ⓑ： reduce a fever   relieve constipation
  help prevent blood clots relieve symptoms of allergies
  prevent motion sickness decrease anxiety
  lower blood pressure reduce high blood cholesterol levels
  promote reduction of lipid levels in the blood
  curb hunger and help you lose weight（空腹を抑えて減量を助ける）

(3) They cause mild/severe side effects. These may include ＿＿＿＿Ⓒ＿＿＿＿.

 Ⓒ： a headache nausea a sick feeling
  sleep problems（睡眠問題 / 障害） restlessness（情動不安）
  bleeding gums（歯茎からの出血） sexual problems
  prolonged nosebleeds（鼻血が止まりにくい）

ⓒ(つづき)：heavy periods in women（生理が重い）   a dry mouth

sleepiness/drowsiness   blurred vision

reduced co-ordination, reaction speed and judgment（調整，反応，判断の遅れ）

Work in Pairs

One partner names the medication from（1）-（2）above. His/her partner tries to explain the adverse effects from（3）above. Change roles.

Example

Ⓐ I am taking pain relievers to reduce a fever.

Ⓑ They make you feel sleepy.

Answers：

Ⓐ _____

Ⓑ _____

10・3 Pronunciation Practice

🔊)) Track 56   ■ Pronounce the following words with special emphasis on accent, rhythm, and stress, etc...

1. blood clot
   [blʌd klɑ́t]

2. hypnotic
   [hipnɑ́tik]

3. tranquilizer
   [trǽŋkwəlàizər]

4. analgesics
   [æ̀nəldʒíːziks]

5. cholesterol
   [kəléstəròul, -rɑːl]

6. vomiting
   [vɑ́mitiŋ]

7. laxative
   [lǽksətiv]

8. anticoagulant
   [æ̀ntaikouǽgjələnt]

9. antipyretics
   [æ̀ntaipairétiks]

10・4 Speak Like a Pharmacist in English

■ Answer the following questions orally in English.

Questions:

1. Tell a patient he doesn't look well.

2. Ask a patient about her other symptoms.

3. Ask a patient if she is on anything now.

4. Ask a patient about her blood pressure.

5. Recommend a patient to see a nearby doctor.

10 · 5   Dictation

■ Listen carefully and write down what is said.

Answers:

1.

2.

3.

4.

5.

6.

7.

8.

10 · 6   Reading Comprehension

 Track 58   ■ Read the following passage within 5 minutes and answer all the questions orally in English.

Severe headaches can have a significant negative impact on quality of life. Many individuals are reluctant to see a doctor, so they go to a pharmacy to seek relief from their headaches. Initial care is provided by a pharmacist, such as choosing an appropriate medication. A headache can sometimes be an indication of something more serious. Therefore, a pharmacist may recommend that a patient see a doctor if their headaches do not improve or worsen with appropriate use of over-the-counter drugs. Examples of a worsening condition include an increase in severity or frequency of headaches, or the addition of a new symptom, such as a high fever, confusion, dizziness, numbness, blurred vision, slurred speech, nausea, or persistent vomiting.

 Track 59   **Questions** (Listen to the recording.)

Answers:

1. _____

2. _____

3. _____

4. _____

5. _____

6. _____

10 · 7   Listening Comprehension

■ Listen carefully and answer all the questions orally in English.   Track 60

Questions:

1. In many cases, which parts of the body are related to coughs caused by common colds?
2. Can cough medicines shorten coughing time or stop a cough?
3. After how long does a cough normally clear up?
4. What should a patient do if they cough up blood?
5. When should a pharmacist tell a patient that they need immediate medical attention?
6. Why should a patient see a doctor if a cough is accompanied by other symptoms?

Answers:

1. _____

2. _____

3. _____

4. _____

5. _____

6. _____

10 · 8   Make Your Own Dialog

■ Based on what you studied in this unit, work with a partner to make a dialog in English between a pharmacist and a patient.

Situation

Listen to the medical history of a patient, ask questions, and finally recommend that she see a doctor.

Answers：

A _____

B _____

A _____

B _____

A _____

B _____

A _____

B _____

COLUMN

受 診 勧 奨

　薬剤師は，薬局に訪れた体調のすぐれない方の訴えなどから，生活指導で十分か，一般用医薬品で対応可能かに続いて，医療機関への受診を促す必要があるのかを鑑別する必要があります．このような分類を行うことを**トリアージ**とよぶこともあります．たとえば"頭が痛い"という患者が薬局に来た場合，頭痛薬を販売すればよいでしょうか？ 答えは No です．激痛が発作的に起こる，といった場合は群発頭痛であったり，頭痛に発熱や吐き気などを伴っていれば髄膜炎といって"細菌"などによって強い炎症を起こしているといったケースも考えられます．このような場合は病院に受診させ，しっかりと治療を受けてもらう必要があります．受診勧奨が必要な場合は病名を当てる必要はありません．患者の全身状態がとても悪いと判断すれば迷わず受診勧奨する姿勢が大切です．

　一方最近，薬局でも簡単な検査ができるようになってきました．血圧や血糖を測ったりすることです．その際，生活指導を続けていても改善がみられなければ病院で薬を出してもらう必要があるかもしれません．こういった場合も受診勧奨が必要になります．薬剤師には地域の患者の健康を担う大切な役割があるのです．　　　　（林　宏行）

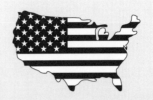

米国に留学して薬剤師になる！
〜 留学準備から臨床薬剤師になるまで 〜

　筆者は，日本で病院薬剤師として勤務した後，米国専門大学院 Pharm.D. 課程に進学した．Pharm.D. 課程修了後はレジデンシー研修を修了し，米国の病院に臨床薬剤師として勤務した．ここでは，米国で薬剤師になる方法，米国の薬学教育・薬剤師業務について紹介する．

1．米国大学の受験システム

　日本の大学における薬学部 6 年制教育が，一般教育・専門教育・研究を一貫して行う学士課程であるのに対し，米国の薬学部は大学院教育であり，入学する時点で学生の多くがすでに何らかの学士号を取得している．大学院は，研究を行う大学院（graduate school：修士・博士課程）と，薬剤師になるための臨床教育を行う専門職大学院（professional school：Pharm.D. 課程）に分かれており，薬剤師免許試験の受験資格が得られるのは Pharm.D. 課程の卒業者のみである．そのため，大学院進学時に将来の方向性を決めていなければならない．同じ Pharm.D. 課程でも大学によって修業年数・入学条件が異なるため，志望校を決定する際は，個々の大学の特徴に加えて，留学生の受験条件・受け入れ実態を調査する必要がある．

2．米国留学に必要な条件

　留学に必要な準備として，満たすべき条件がおもに三つある．一つは学費である．Pharm.D. 課程は 4 年制であり，学費だけで年間 400〜600 万円を要する．数は少ないものの，3 年制の大学や，外国人薬剤師を対象にした 2 年半程度のコースを設置している大学もあり，これらの大学を選択すれば，在学期間を短縮することにより生活費を抑えられるメリットがある．次に，十分な英語力が必要である．Pharm.D. 留学の場合，1 年次から病院・薬局での実務研修を行うプログラムも多く，高いコミュニケーション能力が求められる．TOEFL（Test of English as a Foreign Language）の PBT 550 点（CBT 213 点）を受験条件の最低ラインとしている大学が多く，実際に授業についていくためには PBT 600 点（CBT 250 点）以上が求められると思っていたほうがよい．最後に，志望校の受験条件を調べ，日本の大学の単位が移行できる科目とできない科目を把握する必要がある．

　筆者の場合，日本の大学の単位だけでは条件を満たせず，特に英語についてはスピーチを含む 3 科目を米国の大学で取得する必要があった．留学資金に余裕がなかったため，日中は薬局で働き，夜間に日本の米軍基地内にあるメリーランド大学ユニバーシティ・カレッジ アジア校（https://www.asia.umuc.edu/）に通って必要単位を取得した．早い時期に同じ条件で受験できる大学を複数選出し，不足単位を補うことが重要である．なお，受験条件の単位を満たすだけでなく，特に科学系科目については成績も重要である．日本の大学の単位を移行する場合，1〜2 年次の一般教養科目の成績が大きく影響することを付け加えておく．

3. 米国で薬剤師になる方法

　日本の薬剤師免許を取得している場合，米国の薬剤師免許を取得する方法は二つある．一つは，FPGEE（Foreign Pharmacy Graduate Equivalency Examination）という外国人薬剤師を対象とした試験に合格し，各州が定めるインターン（実務実習）を修了すること，もう一つは，Pharm.D. 課程を卒業することである．

　FPGEE は，基礎生物化学，薬学，臨床科学分野等から出題される CBT（computer based test）である．この FPGEE に合格し，TOEFL の PBT 550 点（CBT 213 点）以上，TSE（スピーキング試験）50 点以上の条件を満たすと，FPGEC（Foreign Pharmacy Graduate Examination Committee）Certification とよばれる薬剤師免許試験の受験資格と薬局・病院での研修資格を得ることができる．FPGEE を選択する場合，日本で受験準備ができて留学費用がかからないが，米国で就職する際に必要な労働ビザの取得が難しい．労働ビザの発給は米国の景気や雇用情勢に左右されるため，外国人の就職は近年厳しくなっている．Pharm.D. 課程への進学を選択する場合は時間と費用を要するが，米国の薬学教育を体験し，臨床薬剤師になるための基礎を築くことができる．"臨床薬剤師"を目指して留学する場合は，Pharm.D. 課程への進学が遠いようで近道である．

4. Pharm.D. 課程における薬学教育

　Pharm.D. 課程に入学すると，学生はインターン免許を取得できる．カリキュラム内の実務研修は"クラークシップ"，カリキュラム外の実務研修は"インターンシップ"とよばれる．薬剤師免許試験の受験資格を得るためには，Pharm.D. 課程を卒業し，州が定める実務研修時間を修了しなければならない．Pharm.D. 課程の最終学年で 1 年間クラークシップを行うが，研修時間の条件を満たせないため，学生の大半は，放課後や週末にインターンシップを行っている．インターンシップのおもな役割は，処方箋の授受と疑義照会，患者の薬歴作成と薬歴調査，調剤，患者および医療関係者からの相談の対応，服薬指導を含む医薬品情報提供である．薬剤師の監督の下では薬剤師同様の仕事が行える．

　Pharm.D. 課程のカリキュラムの魅力は，薬剤師による薬物療法の講義とクラークシップである．日本の大学では 5 カ月間の実務実習を行っているが，米国では 1〜2 年間で 1 実習 4〜6 週間の臨床研修を複数選択する．急性期治療，薬局，薬剤師外来などの必修実習に加え，選択実習として，長期ケア・老年学・在宅治療・小児科・小児 ICU（intensive care unit）・循環器・医薬品情報・薬物動態・核薬学・がん・栄養学・ICU・薬局管理・感染症・HIV（human immunodeficiency virus）・臨床研究・海外研修などのなかから複数選択することができ，とても幅広い．このように，学生はさまざまな実習を経験し，卒業後は病院や薬局に就職して現場の即戦力になる．

5. 米国の臨床薬剤師業務

　米国の病院では，日本のような新卒一括採用は一般的にしないため，就職先を探す際は薬剤師

経験者とポストを競うことになる．近年，Pharm.D. 課程を卒業するだけでは“臨床薬剤師”の職には就けなくなってきており，“レジデンシーを修了していることが望ましい”と条件を付けた募集が増加している．レジデンシーとは，臨床薬剤師になるための卒後トレーニングのことである．

　日本と米国の薬剤師の大きな違いは，米国の薬剤師には“プロトコール型処方権”があることである．プロトコールとは，“定められた条件の下，薬剤師に処方権を委譲することを文書化した計画”のことをいい，共同業務を行う医師－薬剤師間の同意書としての役割を果たしている．薬剤師が処方できる薬剤には，ワルファリン，バンコマイシン，アミノグリコシド系抗菌薬，抗がん剤治療における制吐薬，腎機能低下時の投与設計などがある．

　米国の臨床薬剤師は，患者の薬物療法管理をプロトコールに従い行っている．たとえば，抗菌薬に関しては，患者のアレルギー歴，身長・体重，抗生剤を使用する理由，腎・肝機能，投与期間，血液培養検査結果，血中濃度測定結果，バイタルサイン，白血球数などをモニタリングし，投与設計を行っている．抗菌薬の使用が不適切な場合，薬剤変更・中止については医師に連絡し，TDM（therapeutic drug monitoring）の結果や腎機能低下に基づく投与量についてはプロトコールに基づき薬剤師が処方を変更できる．米国では薬剤師がプロトコール型処方や薬物療法のモニタリングを行うことにより，薬の医療事故を未然に防ぐ手助けをしているだけでなく，医師が患者の診療により専念できる環境づくりにも貢献している．

6. 国際社会における日本の薬剤師の役割——日本から世界に向けて

　近年，日本ではグローバル人材育成が課題となっている．“グローバル人材”と聞くと，語学力やコミュニケーション力が高い人材を思い浮かべるかもしれないが，強みはそれだけではない．主体的かつ積極的に物事に取組む能力，チャレンジ精神，異文化理解と柔軟な対応能力，多様な人々との協調性など幅広い．薬剤師として留学経験があることの強みは，海外で学んだことを日本の薬学教育や薬剤師実務に活かせることに加え，日米の薬学教育，薬剤師業務の違いやその背景，おのおのの長所と短所を理解したうえで問題を評価したり，情報交換・発信ができたりすることである．海外の薬学関係者と交流することにより，海外から見た日本についても情報収集することができる．日本の薬剤師は，自然災害，高齢化社会への対応など，海外の薬剤師が情報を必要としている領域での経験が豊富である．一人でも多くの薬学生に，日本だけでなく，世界の医療に貢献できる薬剤師を目指してもらいたい．

　最後に，留学する際は，最終的に働く場所が米国なのか，日本なのかを考えておくべきである．さらに，留学目的をはっきりさせておくとよい．自己研鑽なのか，日本で専門家不足の領域を学んで先駆者を目指すのか，その目的によって留学中に学ぶべきことが異なってくる．臨床薬学に限らず，医療経済，レギュラトリーサイエンス，医療 IT など，日本でグローバル人材が不足している領域は数多い．これから留学するのであれば，自分自身の興味はもちろん重要であるが，日本で専門家が少ない領域を学んで持ち帰り，日本の薬学発展のために尽力してもらえたら嬉しく思う．

（岩澤真紀子）

PART Ⅲ

Hospital

UNIT 11

Patient Interview

誤解は不適切な薬物療法につながるため，薬剤師が患者と効果的にコミュニケーションをとることは，ファーマシューティカルケアの実践においてとても重要である．

薬剤師は調剤する前に，アレルギー歴，喫煙や飲酒などの生活習慣，服用薬に関する情報を患者から得なければならない．アレルギー反応と副作用を区別することが難しいこともあるため，薬剤師はアレルギーの可能性を判断するために必要な情報を，患者からできるだけ収集する必要がある．

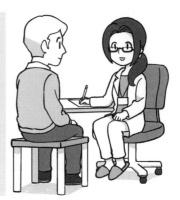

11・1　Dialog

■ Listen to the dialog and memorize it.

🔊 Track 61

薬 Hello, Mr. Smith. How are you?

患 I am all right.

薬 I am glad to hear that. I am your pharmacist, Suzuki. Since this is my first time to see you, would you mind if I ask you about your medication history?

患 No, not at all.

薬 Do you have any food or drug allergies?

患 Yes, I had an allergic reaction to a drug when I was young.

薬 Can you tell me the name of the drug?

患 No, I cannot. It happened more than 20 years ago.

薬 What happened when you took that medication?

患 I had a pretty bad skin rash on both arms.

rash　発疹

薬 OK. Do you smoke?

患 No, I don't.

薬 Do you drink?

患 Yes, I do.

薬 How often? What and how much do you drink?

患 I drink a can of beer almost every day before dinner.

薬 Are you taking any medications now?

患 No.

薬 Thank you for your time.

11・2 Useful Expressions

■ Let's learn how to describe *drug efficacy and side effects*:   ② Specific medicine

(1) This is/these are _____Ⓐ_____.

Ⓐ: antibiotics（抗生物質）   cold medicines（かぜ薬）
    a cough syrup（咳止めシロップ）   antidiarrheals（下痢止め）
    antinauseants/antiemetics（鎮吐薬）   diuretics/water pills（利尿薬）
    stomach medicines（胃薬）   a compress（湿布）
    antitussives/cough suppressants/cough medicines（鎮咳薬）
    antipruritics/anti-itching medications（止痒薬）

(2) They are medicines that _____Ⓑ_____.

Ⓑ: relieve coughs/itching/pain   relieve symptoms of a cold
    prevent nausea   treat severe diarrhea
    suppress airway/trachea/bronchi inflammation（気道 / 気管 / 気管支
        の炎症を抑える）
    reduce the amount of water in the body by increasing the flow of
        urine（排尿を促進し体内の水分を減らす）

(3) They cause mild/severe side effects. These may make you
    have_____Ⓒ_____.

Ⓒ: a headache   nausea   a sick feeling
    sleepiness/drowsiness   blurred vision
    a poor appetite（食欲不振）   stomach irritation（胃痛）
    a dry mouth（口渇）   a dry throat（喉の渇き）
    reduced coordination, reaction speed and judgment（調整，反応，判
        断の遅れ）

Work in Pairs

One partner names the medication from (1) − (2) on page 88. His/her partner tries to explain the adverse effects from (3) on page 88. Change roles.

Example

A I am taking a non-drowsy cold medicine.

B This medicine may make you have a dry throat.

Answers：

A _____

B _____

11 · 3　Pronunciation Practice

■ Pronounce the following words with special emphasis on accent, rhythm, and stress, etc...) Track 62

1. allergic
   [əláːrdʒik]

2. penicillin
   [pènəsílin]

3. bronchitis
   [braŋkáitis]

4. diuretics
   [dàiərétiks]

5. alkane
   [ǽlkein]

6. rheumatism
   [rúːmətìzm]

7. compound
   [kámpaund]
   （名詞）化合物

8. trachea
   [tréikiə]

9. artery
   [áːrtəri]

11 · 4　Speak Like a Pharmacist in English

■ Answer the following questions orally in English.

Questions：

1. Introduce yourself to a patient in a hospital setting.

2. Politely ask to take a medical history.

_____

3. Ask about allergies to food or drugs.

_____

4. Ask questions about the patient's lifestyle.

_____

5. What should you always say after taking a medical history?

_____

11·5 Dictation

Track 63 ■ Listen carefully and write down what is said.

Answers:

1. _____

2. _____

3. _____

4. _____

5. _____

6. _____

7. _____

8. _____

11 · 6   Reading Comprehension

■ Read the following passage within 5 minutes and answer all the questions Track 64
orally in English.

Pharmacists cannot diagnose medical conditions. But they can answer many questions about medicines, recommend nonprescription drugs, and discuss side effects of specific medicines. And some also can provide blood sugar and blood pressure monitoring and offer advice on home monitoring tests.

Most pharmacists who graduated in the 1980s received 5-year bachelor's degrees. It has become the standard for pharmacists to receive a doctor of pharmacy degree. This 6- to 8-year program requires pharmacists in training to go on hospital rounds with doctors and be there when decisions are made to begin medicine use. After getting their degrees, many pharmacists get additional residency training so they can work in a hospital setting.

Pharmacists are required to stay updated on the changing world of medicine and to take continuing education classes on drug therapy.

出 典: Elora Hilmas, *Talking to the Pharmacist*, KidsHealth のウエブサイト〔https://
kidshealth.org/en/parents/pharmacist.html?ref=search（2019 年 11 月現在）〕より転載.
©1995−2019. The Nemours Foundation/KidsHealth®. All Rights Reserved.

Questions（Listen to the recording.） Track 65

Answers:

1. _____

2. _____

3. _____

4. _____

5. _____

6. _____

---

11 · 7 **Listening Comprehension**

 Track 66   ■ Listen carefully and answer all the questions orally in English.

Questions:

1. What two things should you tell your pharmacist about your child?
2. What should you do when you get your meds?
3. When checking even a refill, what three things should you look for?
4. What are two options mentioned for storing a medicine?
5. What are three questions you should ask about giving your child medicines?
6. Lastly, what should you always remember to do?

Answers:

1. _____

2. _____

3. _____

4. _____

5. _____

6. _____

---

11 · 8 **Make Your Own Dialog**

■ Based on what you studied in this unit, work with a partner to make a dialog in English between a pharmacist and a patient.

Situation

You visited Mr. Smith for an initial interview. He had breathing problems after taking his medication in the past. Ask him as many questions as you can to obtain information regarding his medication allergies.

Answers：

A _____

B _____

A _____

B _____

A _____

B _____

A _____

B _____

COLUMN　　　　　病院薬剤師の責務

　病院薬剤師として勤務していた時代のことですが，当時は自ら担当する病棟の薬剤業務を行いながら，病棟薬剤師全体を管理する仕事も担っていました．あるとき，小児科から病棟薬剤業務の依頼がありました．親が子供の使用している薬剤の情報などについて詳しく知りたいというのが依頼理由でした．私は深く考えることなく，病棟薬剤師チームに配属された新人の薬剤師を担当にしました．ほどなくして患児の親から担当薬剤師を交代させてほしいとのクレームがありました．患児の親と担当していた薬剤師の双方から詳しく事情を聞いてみると，患児の親の薬物療法に関する質問に対して，薬剤師が満足に返答できないというのがその理由でした．

　当たり前のことではありますが，患児の親は自分の子供の疾病の治療に懸命です．文献やインターネット，治療の会などのネットワークなどで広範で詳細な知識や情報をもっているのです．ところが，新人薬剤師は経験や知識が乏しく，満足な回答やアドバイスができないのでした．医療人たる者，その道の専門家として常に最新で深い知識をもっていなければならないことを痛感させる事例でした．

（岸川幸生）

UNIT 12

Medicine Brought from Home

患者が家から持参した薬（持参薬）について，薬剤名，用法用量，投薬期間，服薬の目的に関する情報を収集することは，薬剤師の役割の一つである．患者の服用薬の全容を把握することは，患者が薬を適切に服用していたかどうかを薬剤師が評価する際に役立つ．患者の入院時や転院時に，服用薬と病院内で新たに処方された薬とを比較し，不一致や潜在的な問題がないかを確認するプロセスのことを，米国では "medication reconciliation" とよんでいる．

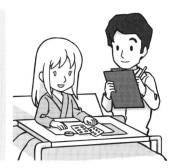

12・1　Dialog

🔊 Track 67　■ Listen to the dialog and memorize it.

薬 Ms. Emma Brown? How are you today? My name is Mori, and I will be your pharmacist in this ward. Do you have time to talk about your medications?

患 Of course.

薬 Do you have your medications with you?

患 Yes, here they are.

medical record handbook　お薬手帳

薬 Do you have your medical record handbook?

患 Yes, here you go.

prescribed　処方された

薬 OK. I will go over your medications with you. It says here that you were prescribed eye drops and two kinds of oral medications. Have you taken the medicines as prescribed?

患 I completed my eye treatment, so I stopped taking the eye drops. I am currently taking two kinds of medications for my blood pressure.

薬 I see. About this white pill, how many times a day have you taken the medication? And when did you take it?

患 I have taken it once a day, after breakfast.

薬 How many tablets do you take at a time?

患 Uh...Two tablets at a time.

薬 How about the other medicine?

患 I take one tablet once a day after breakfast.

薬 I see. Are you currently taking any over-the-counter drugs or supplements?

患 No, I'm not.

薬 I see. Thank you for your help.

12・2   Useful Expressions

■ Let's learn how to describe *allergies*:

(1) I have a/an _____Ⓐ_____allergy. / I'm allergic to _____Ⓐ_____.

Ⓐ: egg/eggs   wheat（小麦）   milk/dairy
    buckwheat（そば）   peanut/peanuts   fish
    shrimp / prawns（えび）   soy beans（大豆）   beef
    shellfish/crab（かに）   pork   chicken   alcohol
    orange/oranges   apple/apples   peach/peaches

(2) The main causes of childhood asthma（小児喘息）are _____Ⓑ_____.

Ⓑ: smoke from cigarettes or fireworks   mold（かび，菌）   stress
    animal fur/dander（動物のふけ，鱗屑）   insect parts   pollen
    viral or other respiratory tract infections
    strenuous exercise（exercise-induced asthma）
    inhaled allergens（dust mite droppings and carcasses, house dust）
    climate or weather conditions（seasonal changes or severe weather
        conditions such as typhoons）

(3) I have _____Ⓒ_____.

Ⓒ *Skin symptoms*: itching   hives（じん麻疹）   reddening（発赤）
    Eye symptoms: itching   redness   swelling of the eyelids
    Digestive symptoms: nausea   abdominal pain   diarrhea
    Oral symptoms: discomfort in the mouth   swelling of the lips
    Respiratory symptoms: a raspy voice（しゃがれ声）   coughing
        wheezing（喘鳴）   difficulty breathing
        a whistling sound（ヒューヒューと鳴る音）when breathing

Ⓒ(つづき)： *Shock symptoms*： loss of consciousness   fatigue（倦怠感）

blue-white lips and/or nails

Nasal symptoms： sneezing   a runny nose

nasal congestion（鼻詰まり）

(4) When I eat them/have it, I become _____Ⓓ_____.

Ⓓ： thirsty   sick   nauseous

(5) When I touch _____Ⓔ_____, I get hives.

Ⓔ： house dust   rubber/latex   pollen

Work in Pairs

One partner asks about allergies. His/her partner tries to name some
from (1) – (5) above. Change roles.

Example
Ⓐ Do you have any allergies?
Ⓑ Yes, I have a buckwheat allergy. When I eat it, I have difficulty
breathing.

Answers：

Ⓐ _____

Ⓑ _____

12・3 Pronunciation Practice

))) Track 68   ■ Pronounce the following words with special emphasis on accent, rhythm,
and stress, etc...

1. ward
    [wɔːrd]

2. record
    [rékərd]

3. digestive
    [daidʒéstiv]

4. vaccination
    [væksənéiʃən]

5. mumps
    [mʌmps]

6. measles
    [míːzlz]

7. rubella
    [ruːbélə]

8. saliva
    [səláivə]

9. muscular dystrophy
    [mʌ́skjulər dístrəfi]

12 · 4   Speak Like a Pharmacist in English

■ Answer the following questions orally in English.

Questions:

1. Ask a patient in a hospital to see her meds from home.

2. Ask to see the patient's medical record handbook.

3. Check to see if the patient has adhered to the prescription.

4. Ask a patient if she is taking any OTC meds or supplements.

5. What is a polite way to end a medical interview?

12 · 5   Dictation

■ Listen carefully and write down what is said.   Track 69

Answers:

1.

2.

3.

4.

5.

6.

7. _____

8. _____

12・6 Reading Comprehension

 Track 70   ■ Read the following passage within 5 minutes and answer all the questions orally in English.

*1 Tylenol（商品名）：アセトアミノフェン製剤・解熱鎮痛薬.

*2 アセトアミノフェン血中濃度が 10〜20 μg/mL の範囲であれば安全と考えられている.

*3 肝機能検査値である GOT，GPT の値が上昇することは，すなわち肝機能障害が疑われる.

A patient with a fever refused the hospital-supplied Tylenol[*1]. The patient's parent brought in the patient's home supply, and the nurse said the child could take that because the fever needed to be treated. The nurse went out to get an oral syringe, and when he came back to the room, the mother said she gave the child what "seemed like a lot of Tylenol." The nurse asked how much, and the parent said 20 mL, which would be 640 mg. The doctor was notified and labs were obtained, which showed an acetaminophen level of 30[*2] and liver functions tests (serum glutamic oxaloacetic transaminase and serum glutamate pyruvate transaminase) increased significantly[*3].

出 典: *Patients Taking Their Own Medications While in the Hospital*, Pennsylvania Patient Safety Authority のウエブサイト〔http://patientsafety.pa.gov/ADVISORIES/documents/201206_50.pdf（2019 年 11 月現在）〕より転載. © 2019 Pennsylvania Patient Safety Authority

 Track 71   **Questions**（Listen to the recording.）

Answers:

1. _____

2. _____

3. _____

4. _____

5. _____

6. _____

12 · 7   Listening Comprehension

■ Listen carefully and answer all the questions orally in English.   )) Track 72

Questions:

1. Who is the intended audience for this announcement?

2. According to the announcement, what are patients asked to do when hospitalized?

3. What types of medications should they bring in?

4. What are strips of tablets?

5. Why does the speaker ask patients to bring in the medication?

6. What is a green bag?

Answers:

1. _____

2. _____

3. _____

4. _____

5. _____

6. _____

12 · 8   Make Your Own Dialog

■ Based on what you studied in this unit, work with a partner to make a dialog in English between a pharmacist and a patient.

Situation

You visited Mr. Jackson for an initial interview. He told you he was taking over-the-counter drugs at home. Ask him as many questions as you can to obtain information regarding the over-the-counter drugs.

Answers：

A

B

A

B

A

B

A

B

COLUMN 持参薬の確認

　2005 年に "入院時患者持参薬に関する薬剤師の対応について" が通達され（日本病院薬剤師会），薬剤師は持参薬の確認・管理に積極的に関与し，患者の安全確保を担うことが望まれています．特に近年，持参薬を入院時に持ち込む患者の比率は高くなっています．加えて，クリニカルパス導入による入院期間の短縮，入院治療費の包括化などが導入され，医療安全と経費節減の両面から，薬剤師による持参薬の確認・管理が強く求められるようになりました．

　持参薬を有する患者の入院時には，薬剤師が面談して医薬品に関する情報収集を行います．医師による処方や医薬品に関する指示出しは，持参薬情報を確認後に行います．また，持参薬の医薬品名，用法用量は，薬袋，診療情報提供書，お薬手帳などで確認しますが，不明の場合は，紹介・処方先の施設に問合わせを行い，持参薬の情報収集に努めています．

　薬剤師が入院早期に持参薬を含めた医薬品情報を収集することで，必然的に薬物療法への介入の機会を得ることができます．さらに，相互作用，重複処方および服薬コンプライアンスを確認することも可能です．これは，医薬品の適正使用への貢献および医療安全を配慮した療養指導につながるため，持参薬の確認・管理に対して薬剤師が果たすべき役割は大きくなっています．

（辻　泰弘）

UNIT 13

Pre-operative Interview

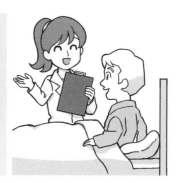

"薬剤師外来"は，日本では比較的新しい薬剤師の臨床業務であり，がん，糖尿病，喘息，循環器（抗凝固薬，心不全）など，さまざまな種類がある．

薬剤師は，薬物療法の効果と安全性を向上させるために，外来患者にファーマシューティカルケアを提供している．たとえば，医薬品のなかには，手術前に服用を中止しなければならないものがある．薬剤師が患者と面談して服用薬の全容を把握し，中止すべき薬について患者に伝えることはとても重要である．

13・1 Dialog

■ Listen to the dialog and memorize it.

🔊)) Track 73

薬 Mr. Wilson, how are you feeling today?

患 I feel good. Thank you.

薬 My name is Sato. I am a pharmacist here in the pre-admission clinic. You will have your surgery next month, won't you?

> pre-admission 入院前

患 Yes. I have never had surgery before, so I am pretty anxious about it.

薬 I know how you feel. Please don't worry.

患 I will try.

薬 So, before you were referred here, did Dr. Suzuki explain about your medications?

患 Yes. He told me that a pharmacist would explain them to me in more detail.

> in more detail さらに詳しく

薬 I see. Although Dr. Suzuki has already asked you similar questions, let me ask you more questions about your medications.

患 No problem.

薬 According to our records, you have never had any allergies or drug side effects. Is this correct?

[患] Yes.

[薬] Are you taking any over-the-counter medicines or supplements in addition to your current prescription medications?

[患] No, I'm not.

[薬] I see. You are taking a medication called warfarin. Since this medication may increase the risk of bleeding, you must stop taking it five days before your surgery.

bleeding 出血

[患] OK. Is there anything else?

[薬] No, that is all. But please let me or Dr. Suzuki know when you start taking any new medications.

[患] I understand. Thank you.

13 · 2   Useful Expressions

■ Let's learn how to describe *medical history*:

(1) I had _____ Ⓐ _____.

    Ⓐ: heart disease（心臓病）   a myocardial infarction（心筋梗塞など）

       angina pectoris（狭心症）   chronic kidney disease（慢性腎臓病）

       kidney failure（腎不全）   a cerebral hemorrhage（脳出血）

       a brain infarction（脳梗塞）   a stroke（脳卒中）   anemia（貧血）

       liver disease（肝臓病）   diabetes（糖尿病）   asthma（喘息）

       gastric or duodenal ulcer（胃・十二指腸潰瘍）

       high blood pressure（高血圧）   hyperlipidemia（高脂血症）

       hyperuricemia（高尿酸血症）   gout（痛風）

       glaucoma（緑内障）   a cataract（白内障）

       prostatic enlargement（前立腺肥大）   epilepsy（てんかん）

(2) I have received _____ Ⓑ _____.

    Ⓑ: dialysis therapy（人工透析）   radiation therapy（放射線療法）

       additional endocrine therapy（追加的内分泌療法）

       chemotherapy for cancer（がん化学療法）

(3) I had _____ Ⓒ _____.

ⓒ：an operation to remove gallstones five years ago（5 年前に胆石を取除
く手術）

my appendix taken out when I was 18（18 歳のときに盲腸を取除いた）

Work in Pairs

One partner asks about the treatment history. His/her partner tries to explain medicinal benefits from (1) – (3) above. Change roles.

Example

Ⓐ Have you ever had surgery before?

Ⓑ I had my appendix taken out when I was 12.

Answers：

Ⓐ _____

Ⓑ _____

13・3　Pronunciation Practice

■ Pronounce the following words with special emphasis on accent, rhythm, and stress, etc...　🔊)) Track 74

1. warfarin
   [wɔ́ːrfərin]

2. hyperlipidemia
   [hàipərlaipidíːmiə]

3. epilepsy
   [épəlèpsi]

4. angina
   [ændʒáinə]

5. cataract
   [kǽtərækt]

6. myocardial
   [màiəkáːrdiəl]

7. anemia
   [əníːmiə]

8. cerebrum
   [səríːbrəm]

9. cerebellum
   [sèrəbéləm]

13・4　Speak Like a Pharmacist in English

■ Answer the following questions orally in English.

Questions：

1. Ask a patient about how he presently feels.

2. Say something to help an anxious patient relax.

_____

3. Reconfirm whether a patient has ever had a drug allergy before.

_____

4. Give a patient a caution when taking warfarin.

_____

5. Remind the patient to talk to you or a doctor if they take a new medication.

_____

13・5 Dictation

 ■ Listen carefully and write down what is said.

Answers:

1. _____

2. _____

3. _____

4. _____

5. _____

6. _____

7. _____

8. _____

13・6 Reading Comprehension

 ■ Read the following passage within 5 minutes and answer all the questions orally in English.

Hospital ambulatory (outpatient) pharmacy has a set of services provided to ambulatory patients, home care patients, hospital staff and probably emergency department patients depending on the level of care of an organization. Ambulatory refers to patients not occupying beds in hospitals or other inpatient settings. Pharmacists play an essential role in the safe, quality and effective use of medications in improving patient's physical and mental wellness. They are instrumental in managing medication-related issues to complement the holistic care for patients throughout the organization. Pharmacists provide education to patients and caregivers on the safe and appropriate use of medications, counsel on medication compliance, monitor and manage medication side effects, as well as screen for dangerous drug interactions.

出 典：E.I.Hammouda, S.E.Hammouda, *Pharmaceut. Reg. Affairs*, 1：101. doi：10.4172/2167-7689.1000101（2012）〔https://www.omicsonline.org/open-access/outpatient-ambulatory-pharmacy-an-innovation-in-dispensing-system-to-optimize-performance-and-meet-standards-2167-7689.1000101.php?aid=5315（2019 年 11 月 現 在 ）〕より転載.

Questions（Listen to the recording.）

Answers：

1. _____

2. _____

3. _____

4. _____

5. _____

6. _____

13・7   Listening Comprehension

◀)) Track 78   ■ Listen carefully and answer all the questions orally in English.

Questions:

1. What are anticoagulant medicines?

2. What can blood clots cause?

3. When do you have to contact the Anticoagulation Team, if you are taking an anticoagulant medicine, and you are planning to become pregnant or are pregnant?

4. Why do you have to immediately contact your Anticoagulation Team if you are planning to become pregnant or are pregnant?

5. Who do you have to consult with if you are taking an anticoagulant medicine and having surgery?

6. What would your Anticoagulation Team do for your surgery?

Answers:

1. _____

2. _____

3. _____

4. _____

5. _____

6. _____

13・8   Make Your Own Dialog

■ Based on what you studied in this unit, work with a partner to make a dialog in English between a pharmacist and a patient.

Situation

　　You visited Mr. Wilson one day after his surgery. Dr. Suzuki told you that he should restart his warfarin on July 1st. Ask him about his condition after the surgery and provide information about restarting the medication.

Answers：

A _____

B _____

A _____

B _____

A _____

B _____

A _____

B _____

COLUMN　　　　**抗がん剤は毒ガス兵器から生まれた**

　ビス（2-クロロエチル）スルフィドを主成分とするマスタードガスはおもにチオジグリコールを塩素化することによって製造される毒ガス兵器として開発されました．ドイツ軍は第一次世界大戦中の 1917 年にイープル戦線で毒ガス兵器として初めて使用します．実戦での特徴的な点として，残留性および浸透性が高いことがあげられ，特にゴムを浸透することが特徴的で，簡単な防護衣では十分な防御が不可能とされています．気化したものは空気よりもかなり重く，低所に停滞し，マスクも対応品が必要です．

　一方，米国も毒ガス兵器としてマスタードガスの硫黄原子を窒素に置き換えたナイトロジェンマスタードを開発しています．1943 年にイタリアのバーリ港に停泊していた連合国の米国海軍輸送船が沈没し，輸送していたマスタードガスが漏れて連合軍兵士は大量に被曝しました．

　被曝者には血圧低下や白血球減少などの症状がみられ，このような症状から当時は X 線照射療法しかなかった悪性リンパ腫の治療が試みられます．その後，ナイトロジェンマスタード誘導体のシクロホスファミドが開発され，現在も血液がんの治療をはじめ広く使用されています．

（中山敏光）

UNIT 14

Chemotherapy

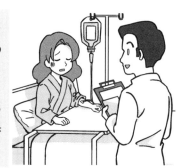

化学療法（chemotherapy）は，臨床現場では"ケモ"と略してよばれることがある．化学療法は，がんを治癒，あるいはがん細胞の広がりを制御し，がんによる痛みや圧迫などの症状を緩和させる．化学療法の後，患者が副作用を経験することはよくあることであり，患者の副作用管理は薬剤師の役割の一つである．がん専門薬剤師（あるいは，がん患者を担当する薬剤師）は，がん治療の安全性，効果および質を確保する責任がある．

14・1　Dialog

))) Track 79　■ Listen to the dialog and memorize it.

薬 Ms. Johnson, how are you today?

患 I feel good, thanks.

薬 My name is Sato, and I will be your pharmacist specializing in oncology. You will start your chemotherapy tomorrow. Did Dr. Tanaka tell you about your premedication schedule before the chemotherapy?

chemotherapy
化学療法

oncology　腫瘍学

premedication
前投薬

患 He told me a pharmacist would explain it in detail to me.

薬 OK.

患 I remember my uncle had chemotherapy and had severe nausea and vomiting after his therapy. I am afraid I will have terrible side effects after the therapy, too.

薬 I know how you feel. It is a fact that some patients experience nausea and vomiting after chemotherapy, so Dr. Tanaka also ordered an anti-nausea medicine to help prevent nausea and vomiting.

患 I see.

薬 Do you have any other questions or concerns?

患 Will my chemotherapy cause hair loss?

薬 It is one of the common side effects, but it depends on the patient. Your hair may start to fall out two to three weeks after starting chemotherapy.

患 When will my hair start to grow back after chemotherapy?

薬 Your hair will start to grow back after your last chemotherapy treatment. By the way, hair that grows back sometimes looks different.

患 I see. I am so nervous.

薬 I will visit you again after your chemotherapy. So if you have any side effects after the therapy, please let me or a nurse know.

患 I will. Thank you.

14・2   Useful Expressions

■ Let's learn how to describe *drug therapies*:

(1) _____ Ⓐ _____ is/are used to _____ Ⓑ _____.

Ⓐ： topical/applied externally steroids（局所用ステロイド薬）and
        tacrolimus ointment（タクロリムス軟膏）

＊括弧内は商品名.

oseltamivir（Tamiflu®）＊oral   aspirin
risedronate（Actonel®）   zolpidem（Ambien®）
insulin glargine（Lantus Solostar Insulin Pen®）
valsartan（Diovan®）   carvedilol（Coreg®）
lansoprazole（Prevacid®）   topiramate（Topamax®）

Ⓑ： control skin inflammation associated with atopic dermatitis
treat symptoms caused by the flu virus（influenza）
reduce fever and relieve mild to moderate pain from conditions such
        as muscle aches, toothaches, the common cold, and headaches
treat a disease that weakens bones
treat a sleep problem/insomnia in adults
control high blood sugar in people with diabetes

Ⓑ(つづき)： treat high blood pressure and heart failure

treat certain stomach and esophagus problems, such as acid reflux, ulcers（胃酸の逆流や潰瘍などの胃・食道障害）

prevent and control seizures/epilepsy（発作 / てんかん）, and prevent migraine headaches（片頭痛）and decrease how often you get them

---

Work in Pairs

One partner names the medication（1-A）above. His/her partner tries to explain the medicinal effects（1-B）above. Change roles.

Example
Ⓐ My doctor prescribed aspirin.
Ⓑ This medicine reduces a fever and relieves mild to moderate pain from conditions such as muscle aches, toothaches, the common cold, and headaches.

Answers：

Ⓐ _____

Ⓑ _____

14・3 Pronunciation Practice

🔊) Track 80 ■ Pronounce the following words with special emphasis on accent, rhythm, and stress, etc...

1. oncology
[ɑŋkálədʒi]

2. chemotherapy
[kìːmouθérəpi]

3. dermatitis
[dɜ̀ːrmətáitis]

4. esophagus
[isáfəgəs]

5. ulcer
[ʌ́lsər]

6. seizure
[síːʒər]

7. hepatitis
[hèpətáitis]

8. nephritis
[nəfráitis]

9. colon cancer
[kóulən kǽnsər]

14・4   Speak Like a Pharmacist in English

■ Answer the following questions orally in English.

Questions:

1. Tell a patient your specialty as a pharmacist.

_____

2. Express empathy to a patient who is worried about drug side effects.

_____

3. Explain that a medicine has been prescribed to help relieve side effects from another medicine.

_____

4. Explain common adverse reactions to chemotherapy.

_____

5. Ask the patient if she has any questions or concerns.

_____

14・5   Dictation

■ Listen carefully and write down what is said.

Answers:

1. _____

2. _____

3. _____

4. _____

5. _____

6. _____

7. _____

8. _____

14・6 Reading Comprehension

 Track 82   ■ Read the following passage within 5 minutes and answer all the questions orally in English.

M.P.H.（Master of Public Health）公衆衛生修士

rampant 蔓延した

bogus 偽の

Beware of products claiming to cure cancer on websites or social media platforms, such as Facebook and Instagram. According to Nicole Kornspan, M.P.H., a consumer safety officer at the U.S. Food and Drug Administration（FDA）, they're rampant these days.

Legitimate medical products such as drugs and devices intended to treat cancer must gain FDA approval or clearance before they are marketed and sold. The agency's review process helps ensure that these products are safe and effective for their intended uses.

Nevertheless, it's always possible to find someone or some company hawking bogus cancer "treatments," which come in many forms, including pills, capsules, powders, creams, teas, oils, and treatment kits. Frequently advertised as "natural" treatments and often falsely labeled as dietary supplements, such products may appear harmless, but may cause harm by delaying or interfering with proven, beneficial treatments. Absent FDA approval or clearance for safety, they could also contain dangerous ingredients.

出 典: *Products Claiming to "Cure" Cancer Are a Cruel Deception*, U.S. FDA のウエブサイト〔https://www.fda.gov/consumers/consumer-updates/products-claiming-cure-cancer-are-cruel-deception（2019 年 11 月現在)〕より転載.

Questions （Listen to the recording.）

Answers:

1. _____

2. _____

3. _____

4. _____

5. _____

---

14 · 7 Listening Comprehension

■ Listen carefully and answer all the questions orally in English.   ))) Track 84

Questions:

1. In the case of bladder cancer, in which part of the body are genetic mutations present?
2. How common is bladder cancer in the United States?
3. What is the approximate percentage of patients with recurrent and refractory bladder cancer who have fibroblast growth factor?
4. How many patients participated in a clinical trial for Balversa?
5. What was the rate of the patients who had a complete response to Balversa?

Answers:

1. _____

2. _____

3. _____

4. _____

5. _____

14・8   Make Your Own Dialog

■ Based on what you studied in this unit, work with a partner to make a dialog in English between a pharmacist and a patient.

> **Situation**
>
> You visited Ms. Johnson after her chemotherapy. Ask about her condition after the chemotherapy. After that, ask her if the medication for nausea and vomiting worked or not.

Answers：

A _____

B _____

A _____

B _____

A _____

B _____

A _____

B _____

COLUMN　　　　　生活と医療を支える不思議なバケツ

　シクロデキストリンはグルコース6〜8個が環状に結合してできたものです．穴のあいたバケツの構造と表現されます．シクロデキストリン自体はヒドロキシ基を多数もつため親水性ではありますが，そのバケツの内側は炭素-炭素結合およびエーテル結合のため疎水性となっているという非常にユニークな特徴をもっています．用途としては水に溶解しにくい疎水性成分をそのバケツの内側で包みこむことで（包接といいます）水と接する部分が親水性であるバケツの外側となります．この結果，水に溶解しやすくなります．

　生活のなかでは消臭剤としての利用があります．消臭剤ではよい匂いの成分をバケツのなかに包接させてあります．不快な臭い成分があるとよい匂いの成分の代わりに不快な臭い成分をバケツの中に包接させることで消臭し，人はよい匂いを感じます．

　医療での応用もあります．体内では臓器が常に緊張した状態となっているため手術などで体を開く際に筋弛緩薬が投与されます．手術終了後もずっと筋弛緩作用が残っていると呼吸ができません．そこでシクロデキストリンの誘導体を体内に投与します．血中の筋弛緩薬をバケツの中に取込むことで筋弛緩効果を消失させます．

（中村公薫）

UNIT 15 Discharge Directions

　病院薬剤師の重要な役割の一つは，退院前に患者を訪れ，退院時の薬について指導することである（日本では薬剤師がこれを行うことにより，"退院時薬剤情報管理指導料"を診療報酬として請求することができる）．薬剤師による退院時指導は，退院時の薬の過誤や副作用を防ぐこと，再入院を減らすこと，服薬アドヒアランスを向上させることが示されている．米国においては，2012年に米国保健社会福祉省のメディケア・メディケイドサービスセンターが"再入院削減プログラム"を開始し，薬剤師による退院患者に対するサービスが拡大している．

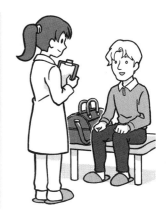

15・1 Dialog

🔊 Track 85　■ Listen to the dialog and memorize it.

薬 Mr. James, how are you today?

患 Pretty good. Thank you.

薬 I heard you will be going home tomorrow.

患 Yes, I am. I am so glad!

薬 I am very pleased to hear that.

appreciate 感謝する

患 I appreciate your kindness during my stay.

薬 You are welcome. Would you mind if I talk to you about your discharge medications now?

患 No, of course not.

edema 浮腫

薬 There are three medications. One medication is furosemide, and this medication helps reduce the symptoms of edema and breathing difficulty. You need to take one tablet after breakfast and lunch.

患 Can I drive a car?

薬 This may cause dizziness or for you to lose your sense of balance. You   dizziness めまい
have to be careful driving.

患 I see.

薬 This medication is called carvedilol. This improves heart failure   heart failure
symptoms and your life prognosis. You need to take one tablet after   心不全
breakfast and dinner.
                                                                      life prognosis
                                                                      生命予後
患 OK.

薬 The last one is candesartan, and you need to take one tablet after
breakfast. This medication will also improve your life prognosis and will
help prevent cardiovascular events. Even if you feel better, do not stop
taking these medications. Do you have any questions?

患 No, I understand.

薬 That's about it. Please take care and feel free to contact me if you have
any questions.

15 · 2   Useful Expressions

■ Let's learn how to describe *symptoms and clinical department names*:

(1) I have _____Ⓐ_____.

Ⓐ: a terrible headache   dizziness   hives（じん麻疹）
     a toothache   a sore arm   an itchy eye
     skin redness   nausea   swelling of the eyelids
     abdominal pain   diarrhea   wheezing（喘鳴）
     a runny nose   coughing   difficulty breathing
     child asthma   sneezing   difficulty sleeping
     a language disorder   a raspy voice（しゃがれ声）
     anxiety（不安神経症）   nasal congestion（鼻詰まり）
     frequent urination   morning sickness（つわり）
     a burn scar（やけど跡）   a broken bone/ fracture of the bone

(2) I sprained my wrist.

（3）Please go to ____Ⓑ____ .

    Ⓑ：internal medicine（内科）   surgery（外科）

         ear, nose and throat（耳鼻咽喉科）   ophthalmology（眼科）

         plastic surgery（形成外科）   orthopedics（整形外科）

         dermatology（皮膚科）   pediatrics（小児科）

         obstetrics and gynecology（産婦人科） urology（泌尿器科）

         dentistry（歯科）   orthodontics（矯正歯科）

         neurosurgery（脳神経外科）   psychiatry（精神科）

         physical therapy（リハビリテーション科） neurology（神経内科）

Work in Pairs

One partner explains the condition from (1)–(2) above. His/her partner tries to suggest the department from (3) above. Change roles.

Example
Ⓐ I have a toothache.
Ⓑ Please go to dentistry.

Answers：

Ⓐ _____

Ⓑ _____

15・3　Pronunciation Practice

 Track 86　■ Pronounce the following words with special emphasis on accent, rhythm, and stress, etc...

1. edema
   [idíːmə]

2. psychiatry
   [saikáiətri]

3. dermatology
   [də̀ːrmətálədʒi]

4. tumor
   [tʲúːmər]

5. prognosis
   [prɑgnóusis]

6. cardiovascular
   [kɑ̀ːrdiouvǽskjulər]

7. obstetrics
   [əbstétriks]

8. ginkgo
   [gíŋkou]

9. pediatrics
   [pìːdiǽtriks]

15 · 4 Speak Like a Pharmacist in English

■ Answer the following questions orally in English.

Questions:

1. Ask when a patient will be discharged.

_____

2. Express happiness at good news.

_____

3. Tell the patient about his discharge medications.

_____

4. Explain a medicine to a patient and tell him the name and purpose of it.

_____

5. End your discharge directions in a polite manner.

_____

15 · 5 Dictation

■ Listen carefully and write down what is said.

Answers:

1. _____

2. _____

3. _____

4. _____

5. _____

6. _____

7. _____

8. _____

15 · 6 Reading Comprehension

 Track 88   ■ Read the following passage within 5 minutes and answer all the questions orally in English.

The role of the Japanese hospital pharmacist has evolved dramatically over the last quarter century. One particularly noteworthy change is our shifted focus from "medication" to "medication management." A decade has passed since the Japanese pharmacy school curriculum transitioned from four-years to six-years. We have always been driven to advance pharmacy practice and improve patient's QOL by applying the principal of pharmaceutical care—safe and effective use of medication. Some of the practices adopted over the years include the participation in team-based medical care in hospital wards, proposition of optimal therapy by performing therapeutic drug monitoring of individual patients, and prevention of adverse drug reactions or significant side effects. We have also initiated a variety of new services such as management of chemotherapy regimens, aseptic preparation of antineoplastic drugs, and the collection and provision of drug information. These accomplishments have made a profound impact on public and patient perception of pharmacist's roles and values. As a result, demand for expanded pharmacist practice sites—at hospitals and clinics, long-term care insurance facilities, and other healthcare facilities—has continued to grow significantly.

出 典: Kenji Kihira, *Message from the President*, Japanese Society of Hospital Pharmacists のウエブサイト〔https://www.jshp.or.jp/gaiyou/pamphlet/pamphlet4.pdf#search=%27hospital+pharmacist%27（2019 年 11 月現在）〕より許可を得て転載. Copyright © 2007–2019 JSHP. All rights reserved.

Questions （Listen to the recording.）

Answers：

1. _____

2. _____

3. _____

4. _____

5. _____

6. _____

15 · 7   Listening Comprehension

■ Listen carefully and answer all the questions orally in English.

Questions：

1. For overseas pharmacists to become hospital pharmacists in the UK, what must they do first?

2. How long is the pre-registration training？

3. What else do you have to pass?

4. When do you have to complete all of the steps?

5. If you are to gain sponsorship from a UK hospital, what else are you required to do?

6. To show your English language competency, what do you have to take?

Answers：

1. _____

2. _____

3. _____

4. _____

5. _____

6. _____

15・8   Make Your Own Dialog

■ Based on what you studied in this unit, work with a partner to make a dialog in English between a pharmacist and a patient.

> **Situation**
>
>   Ms. Brown is going to be discharged. Since she has dementia, you need to talk to her daughter regarding her discharge medications.

Answers:

A _____

B _____

A _____

B _____

A _____

B _____

A _____

B _____

COLUMN　臨床で汎用される略語

どの世界にもその分野に携わる者なら誰でも知っている共通の言葉（業界用語）があります．以下に，臨床で汎用される略語を記します．元々は北米で使われる略語です．これらは医療における職種の枠組みを超えて各種書類，カルテを含めた記録に出てくるので慣れておくとよいでしょう．

症状（symptom）は Sx, 病歴（history）は Hx, 治療（treatment）は Tx, 診断（diagnosis）は Dx, 処方（recipe）または処方箋（prescription）は Rx です（日本では Rp とすることも多い）．骨折（fracture）は Fx.

検査では血算（complete blood counts）は CBC, 肝機能検査（liver function test）は LFT, 血糖（blood sugar）は BS, 心電図（electrocardiogram）は ECG です．

その他，S/O（suspected of, suggestive of, or suspicious of）は "〜の疑い"，R/O（rule out）は "鑑別診断"，F/U（follow up）は "経過を追う" の意味で使われます．また，Do or do（ditto）も "同じ" の意味で汎用されます．たとえば "Do 処方で" のように．

その一方，たとえば DM は糖尿病（diabetes mellitus）の略語と思いがちですが，皮膚筋炎（dermatomyositis）の意味で使うこともあります．

共通の略語以外の使用は誤解を招き，incident and/or accident につながるので，その使用には特段の注意を要します．なお，これらの略語を患者向けの文章・書類に使わないことは言うまでもありません．　　　　　　　　　（小野真一）

付表　米国と英国で一般名の異なる医薬品

国際一般名（INN：International Nonproprietary Name）設定（1950 年）以前に命名された医薬品は米国一般名（USAN：United States adopted name）と英国一般名（BAN：British approved name）で大きな違いがあった．さらに BAN ではヨーロッパの法律に準拠するため一部が INN に変更されたため，USAN と BAN で異なることになったものもある．下表におもな例を記す．

近年の新薬については USAN も BAN も INN に合わせている．

表　米国と英国で一般名の異なる医薬品 [a), †]（＊は INN）

米国一般名（USAN）	英国一般名（BAN）	米国一般名（USAN）	英国一般名（BAN）
acetaminophen	paracetamol*	indomethacin	indometacin*
acyclovir	aciclovir*	isoproterenol	isoprenaline*
albuterol	salbutamol*	leucovorin/ 　leucovorin calcium	folinic acid/ 　calcium folinate
amphetamine	amfetamine*	mechlorethamine	chlormethine 　（mustine）
anthralin	dithranol*	meperidine	pethidine*
apazone	azapropazone*	metaproterenol	orciprenaline*
beclomethasone	beclometasone*	methotrimeprazine/ 　levomepromazine [†, *]	levomepromazine*
cephalexin	cefalexin*	mineral oil	liquid paraffin
cephradine	cefradine*	nafronyl	naftidrofuryl*
chlorpheniramine	chlorphenamine*	niacin	nicotinic acid*
chlorthalidone	chlortalidone*	niacinamide	nicotinamide*
cholestyramine	colestyramine*	nitroglycerin	glyceryl trinitrate
clomiphene	clomifene*	norethindrone	norethisterone*
cosyntropin	tetracosactide* 　（tetracosactrin）	penicillin G	benzylpenicillin*
cromolyn sodium	sodium cromoglicate	penicillin V	phenoxymethylpenicillin*
cyclosporine	ciclosporin*	phytonadione	phytomenadione*
deferoxamine	desferrioxamine	pizotyline	pizotifen*
dextroamphetamine	dexamfetamine*	polyethylene glycols	macrogols
dextrose	glucose	pramoxine	pramocaine*
dicyclomine	dicycloverine*	propoxyphene	dextropropoxyphene*
divalproex sodium	semisodium valproate*	psyllium	ispaghula
epinephrine*	adrenaline/ 　epinephrine*	quinacrine	mepacrine*
ergonovine	ergometrine*	rifampin	rifampicin*
estrogen	oestrogen	scopolamine*	hyoscine
floxacillin	flucloxacillin*	simethicone	simeticone
glutaral*	glutaraldehyde	succinylcholine	suxamethonium*
glyburide	glibenclamide*	sulfamethazine	sulfadimidine*
glycopyrrolate	glycopyrronium bromide*	trimeprazine	alimemazine*
gold sodium thiomalate	sodium aurothiomalate	valacyclovir	valaciclovir*
hydroxyurea	hydroxycarbamide*	valproate sodium	sodium valproate*

a)　*What are the differences between US and UK drug names?*，NHS のウエブサイト〔https://www.sps.nhs.uk/articles/what-are-the-differences-between-us-and-uk-drug-names/（2019 年 11 月現在）〕より一部改変．Copyright © Crown copyright.

†　levomepromazine は，米国薬局方および米国の参考文献で methotrimeprazine としてリストされているが，米国での一般名は levomepromazine であり，文献検索には両方の名前を使用することが必要な場合がある．

かね　こ　とし　お
金 子 利 雄

1956 年 埼玉県生まれ
1980 年 日本大学文理学部英文学科修士課程 修了
1984 年 米国ボール州立大学大学院英語科修士課程 修了
現 日本大学薬学部 教授
専門 英語学
文学修士，M.A.(英語学)

エリック　　　　スカイヤー
Eric M. Skier

1969 年 米国ロサンゼルス生まれ
1991 年 米国国際大学 卒
2002 年 米国コロンビア大学ティーチャーズカレッジ
修士課程 修了
現 日本大学薬学部 准教授
専門 英語教授法
M.A.(英語教授法)

第 1 版 第 1 刷 2021 年 2 月 12 日 発行

薬学生のための英語会話
ー音声データダウンロードサービス付ー

© 2 0 2 1

編　者　　　金 子 利 雄
　　　　　　Eric M. Skier
発 行 者　　　住 田 六 連
発　行　株式会社 東京化学同人
東京都文京区千石 3 丁目 36-7(〒112-0011)
電 話 03-3946-5311・FAX 03-3946-5317
URL: http://www.tkd-pbl.com/

印 刷　日本ハイコム株式会社
製 本　株式会社 松岳社

ISBN978-4-8079-0978-0
Printed in Japan

薬学生・薬剤師のための
英会話ハンドブック 第2版

原　博・Eric M. Skier・渡辺朋子 著

新書判　2色刷　256 ページ　本体 2700 円＋税

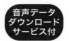

薬局や病院で薬剤師が，英語圏の患者に対応するときに役立つ実践的な英会話集．OTC薬の販売，受診勧奨，服薬指導，病棟での治療薬の説明など実際の場面に沿った会話例を豊富に収載．ネイティブスピーカーにより収録された全ダイアログの音声データダウンロードサービス付．

プライマリー薬学シリーズ 1
薬 学 英 語 入 門

日本薬学会 編　**CD付**

B5 判　144 ページ　本体 2800 円＋税

日本薬学会の薬学教育カリキュラムを検討する協議会が定めた"薬学準備教育ガイドライン"に準拠した薬学生のための英語の教科書．

実 用 薬 学 英 語

日本薬学会 編

B5 判　128 ページ　本体 2200 円＋税

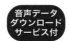

6年制薬学部で学ぶ2, 3年生のための英語の教科書．コアカリキュラム改訂の理念と基本方針にそって，薬剤師としての倫理観，社会性，科学を基盤として医療に貢献できる臨床の力が強く求められていることを反映させるため，モデル・コアカリキュラムの一般目標から偏りなくテーマを選び，各章の英文素材とした．

薬学生のための **実践英語**

Eric M. Skier・上鶴重美 著　**CD付**

A5 判　96 ページ　本体 1600 円＋税

海外研修への参加，英語での学会発表，就職活動などを始めようとしている薬学部の学生向け教科書．口頭や書面での自己紹介の仕方や面接の受け方，メールや履歴書の書き方，プレゼンテーションのコツなどを幅広く紹介する．

2021 年 2 月現在

——— 日本薬学会編 ———

スタンダード薬学シリーズⅡ

全9巻 26冊

総監修 市 川 厚

編集委員 赤池昭紀・伊藤 喬・入江徹美・太田 茂
奥 直人・鈴木 匡・中村明弘

電子版 教科書採用に限り電子版対応可. 詳細は東京化学同人営業部まで.

1 薬 学 総 論
編集責任: 中村明弘

Ⅰ. 薬剤師としての基本事項 4800 円

Ⅱ. 薬学と社会 4500 円

2 物 理 系 薬 学
編集責任: 入江徹美

Ⅰ. 物質の物理的性質 4900 円

Ⅱ. 化学物質の分析 4900 円

Ⅲ. 機器分析・構造決定 4200 円

3 化 学 系 薬 学
編集責任: 伊藤 喬

Ⅰ. 化学物質の性質と反応 5600 円

Ⅱ. 生体分子・医薬品の
化学による理解 4600 円

Ⅲ. 自然が生み出す薬物 4800 円

4 生 物 系 薬 学
編集責任: 奥 直人

Ⅰ. 生命現象の基礎 5200 円

Ⅱ. 人体の成り立ちと
生体機能の調節 4000 円

Ⅲ. 生体防御と微生物 4900 円

5 衛 生 薬 学 —健康と環境—
6100 円
編集責任: 太田 茂

6 医 療 薬 学

Ⅰ. 薬の作用と体の変化および
薬理・病態・薬物治療（1） 4100 円

Ⅱ. 薬理・病態・薬物治療（2） 3800 円
Ⅰ・Ⅱ 編集責任: 赤池昭紀

Ⅲ. 薬理・病態・薬物治療（3） 3400 円

Ⅳ. 薬理・病態・薬物治療（4） 5500 円
Ⅲ・Ⅳ 編集責任: 山元俊憲

Ⅴ. 薬物治療に役立つ情報 4200 円

Ⅵ. 薬の生体内運命 3200 円

Ⅶ. 製剤化のサイエンス 3500 円
Ⅴ・Ⅵ・Ⅶ 編集責任: 望月眞弓

7 臨 床 薬 学
日本薬学会・日本薬剤師会
日本病院薬剤師会・日本医療薬学会 共編
編集責任: 鈴 木 匡

Ⅰ. 臨床薬学の基礎および
処方箋に基づく調剤 4000 円

Ⅱ. 薬物療法の実践 2500 円

Ⅲ. チーム医療および
地域の保健・医療・福祉への参画 4000 円

8 薬 学 研 究
2900 円
編集責任: 市 川 厚

9 薬 学 演 習
—アクティブラーニング課題付—

Ⅰ. 医療薬学・臨床薬学 3400 円
編集責任: 赤池昭紀

Ⅱ. 基 礎 科 学 編集責任: 市 川 厚
2021 年6月刊行予定

Ⅲ. 薬学総論・衛生薬学 3800 円
編集責任: 太 田 茂

記載の価格は本体価格, 定価は本体価格＋税(2021 年2月現在)